No-Cook and Gluten-Free

The Gluten-Free, Dairy Free, No-Cook
Playbook for Every Occasion

Table of Contents

Introduction

Breakfast Recipes

Nutty Oatmeal Bowl

Turkey Jerky Bacon

Crêpes with Cashew Lemon Curd

Lox and Avocado Crêpes

Bananarama Pancake Stack

Coconut Pancakes and Berry Jam

Superfood Breakfast Brownies

Coconut Cake Breakfast Plate

Carrot Biscuits with Sweet Tahini

Lunch Recipes

Mexican Tomato Soup

Carrot Ginger Soup

Tomato Basil Soup

Texas Chili

Creamy "Cheese" and Broccoli Soup

Raspberry Almond Salad

Caesar Salad

Spiced Walnut Autumn Salad

Blueberry Poppy Seed Salad

Pecan Apricot Spinach Salad

Smoked Salmon Avocado Salad

Avocado Persimmon Salad

Sweet Guava Salad

Cocoa Banana Salad

Coconut Beet Salad

Thai Coconut Curry

Banana Cashew Curry

Pesto Tomato Caprese

Cilantro Taco Salad

Asian Shrimp Lettuce Wraps

Savory Stuffed Peppers

Veggie Noodle Pad Thai

Sweet Coconut Waldorf Salad

Fresh Sashimi Bento Bowl

Fresh Clams with Cocktail Sauce

Dinner Recipes

Zucchini Pasta with Sundried Tomato Sauce

Zucchini Pasta with Pesto

Zucchini Fettuccini Alfredo

Cashew Crunch Kelp Noodle Salad

Tuna Tartar with Avocado and Mango

Raw Walnuts Tacos

Tilapia Lettuce Wraps

Butternut Squash Soup

Creamy Pumpkin Soup

City Clam Chowder

Creamy French Onion Soup

Salmon Tartar Stack

Simple Steak Tartar

Beef Carpaccio with Arugula Salad

Spinach Salad with Shallot Vinaigrette

Awesome Oysters

Dill Stuffed Tomatoes

Savory Stuffed Portobello

Garlic Almond Bread

Gyro Wrap with Avocado Tzatziki

Savory Nut Meatloaf

Tuscan Rustic Pizza

Zucchini Mac and Cashew Cheese

Squash Blossom Stuffers

Zucchini Walnut Lasagna

Dessert Recipes

Sweet Banana Cream pie

Creamy Chocolate Pie

Lemon Chiffon Pie

Key Lime Cream Pie

Coconut Cream Pie

Simple Pecan Pie

Modern Mincemeat Pie

Holiday Pumpkin Pie

Creamy Strawberry Cheesecake

Lemon Curd Dessert Tart

Easy Apricot Pie

Blue Ribbon Apple Pie

Perfect Peach Pie

1st Prize Cherry Pie

Fruity Blueberry Pie

Refrigerator Carrot Cake

Tasty Chocolate Cake

New Country Red Velvet Cake

Sweet Treat Banana Bread

Scrumptious Coconut Macaroons

Dunkable Chocolate Chunk Cookies

Dehydrated Almond Biscotti

Ginger Punch Pudding

Creamy Strawberry Ice Cream

Tropical Sorbet

Smoothies Recipes

Homemade Almond Milk

Homemade Coconut Milk

Shredded Coconut Milk

Green Supreme Smoothie

Sweet Envy Green Smoothie

Perfect Pear Smoothie

Red Rave Smoothie

Strawberry Banana Blend

Tropical Colada Mombata

Kiwi Strawberry Smoothie

Peter Rabbit Carrot Crush

Chocolate Banana Shake

Cucumber Melon Slushy

Sweet Strawberry Slushy

Sweet Berry Bliss

Indigo Blue Berry Blend

Nutty Buddy Banana Smoothie

Bright & Early Orange Whirl

Sweet Mango Swirl

Strawberry Orange Smoothie

Sweet Avocado Swirl

Watermelon Cooler Crush

Bananarama Blend

Peach Relief Smoothie

Morning Mellow Melon

Guava Pop Smoothie

Lemon Freeze

Mojito Cooler Crush

On the Go Recipes

Lemon Energy Bars

Ginger Crisps

Crisp Cocoa Wafers

Good Morning Trail Mix

Preserved Beef Jerky

Fruit and Nut Apricot Pockets

Sweet Treat Blondie Bars

Summer Sweet Bread

Coconut Lemon Biscuits

Spicy Sesame Crackers

Cheesy Kale Crisps_

Spicy Jalapeño Poppers

Savory Pepperdew Poppers

Fruity Granola Bars

Banana Berry Fruit Rolls

Crispy Carrot Chips

Acorn Squash Crisps

Confetti Beet Chips

Mango Snacks

Pineapple Chews

Banana Crisps

Sweet Apple Chips

Spicy Kale Crisps

Savory Sweet Potato Chips

Cheesy Popcorn

Kids Recipes

Easy Chocolate Milk

Stuffed Apple Snack

Cashew Cream and Carrots

Chocolate Spread on Celery

Cashew Apple Stack

Simple Banana Pudding

True Chocolate Pudding

Afterschool Applesauce

Almond Butter and Jelly Bars

Pecan Brownies

Chocolate Chip Cookie Dough Bites

Super Fruit Granola Bars

Awesome Chocolate Fudge

Strawberry Fruit Rolls

Chocolate Banana Pops

Orange Cream Popsicles

Sweet Coconut Ice Cream

Lemonade Slush

Cherry Crush

Sweet Potato Sticks

Crispy Onion Rings

Cauliflower Popcorn

Zucchini Lasagna Roll Ups

Squash Blossom Poppers

Meatballs and Tomato Sauce

Snacks Recipes

Crisp Sesame Crackers

Veggie Flax Crackers

Avocado Cashew Hummus with Cucumber

Sundried Tomato Cashew Hummus with Carrots

Cocoa Date Spread

Cashew Spinach Dip with Bell Pepper

Chocolate Hazelnut Spread with Apples

Cashew Butter Date Snacks

Very Cherry Energy Bars

Sweet Coconut Ambrosia Salad

Sweet Carrot Raisin Salad

Sweet Coconut Rice with Mango

Sweet Almond Crunch Cookies

Chewy Ginger Cookies

Chocolate Dusted Almonds

Chocolate Chia Pudding

Coconut Rice Pudding

Nori with Almond Cheese

Quick Asian Slaw

Awesome Strawberry Salsa

Supreme Mango Salsa

Hot Apricot Pineapple Salsa

Fresh Zesty Pico de Gallo

Holy Loaded Guacamole

Spicy Stuffed Jalapeños

Why Gluten-Free, No Cook & Dairy-Free?

In an era of fast-food and processed ingredients, more and more people are seeking to return to a more primal, natural lifestyle. Indeed, it is becoming widely accepted that our modern way of eating is contributing to an epidemic of obesity and auto-immune diseases. The convenience of drive-thrus and microwaves is taking its toll in the form of cancer, fatigue, diabetes, chronic inflammation and heart disease. But just how can a cleaner, raw diet really help us experience improved health and greater energy?

Cooking food has been around for quite some time. In fact, evidence suggests that primitive man started cooking food about 250,000 years ago. While we don't exactly know why our ancestors began cooking their meat, theories suggest that it was discovered by accident or as the result of experimentation. Today, a large portion of our diet is made up of foods that are heated at high temperatures. However, new beliefs are starting to emerge regarding the cooking of food and its detriments to human health.

We are still the only species to cook our food on purpose. Whether it's frying, barbecuing, boiling or microwaving our culinary creations, most of us regard it as a necessity. We have grown to enjoy the taste of cooked meat and veggies, baked fruit pies, bread and coffee. Yet, cooking food changes its chemical structure and destroys the enzymes that help with digestion. Heating foods to high temperatures also destroys some of their nutrients and changes the structure of proteins.

Recent discoveries in the field of nutrition show that heating food produces very damaging by-products known as glycotoxins. According to these findings, glycotoxins contribute to oxidation, premature aging and the onset of chronic inflammation. As we now know, many modern diseases such as dementia, cancer and diabetes are, in fact, directly related to inflammation. New studies suggest that cutting back on cooked foods might help restore the body's natural defenses against disease and inflammation.

Another issue with our modern diet is the over-consumption of certain proteins that our bodies are not designed to digest properly. Anything that isn't properly digested leaks through the small intestine and creates inflammation as the body attempts to fight off a perceived aggression. Two widely-consumed proteins are known to be particularly difficult to digest for most humans: gluten and casein. Gluten is found in grains such as barley, rye and wheat. In about 1% of people, gluten causes a severe auto-immune reaction during which the body attacks its own intestines in the presence of gluten. This condition is known as Celiac Disease. However, new estimates show that not only are most Celiacs still undiagnosed, but as much as 20 to 30% of the population suffers from a less dramatic form of gluten intolerance.

Food intolerances do not always cause digestive distress. In fact, most people who are intolerant to gluten will have more subtle reactions that are seemingly unrelated: worn-out tooth enamel, osteoporosis, anemia, unexplained rashes, fatigue, chronic pain, infertility and difficulties concentrating are only some of the possible symptoms that people don't usually attribute to their morning toast.

Much in the same way, intolerance to casein is thought to be extremely common but few people are aware of its consequences. Casein is found in dairy products such as milk, cheese and yogurt. Casein intolerance is caused by the protein in dairy, while lactose intolerance is caused by its sugar content. Both casein and lactose intolerances often go hand in hand with gluten intolerance. The digestive issues caused by gluten inhibit the production of lactase, the enzyme needed to break down lactose. As such, lactose intolerance is often more of a symptom of another underlying condition.

Many theories exist regarding human evolution and our ability to adapt to a completely new lifestyle. Since agriculture became the preferred method of sustaining our food supply, our diet has shifted from a hunter-gatherer perspective to a more modern, grain-based way of eating. Experts believe that the 10,000 years that have elapsed since the agricultural revolution are far from enough for our bodies to adapt when compared to the timeline of our species' evolution. Primitive man didn't have access to grains and dairy, and it is now thought that our bodies are not actually capable of processing these nutrients properly, leading to fatigue, inflammation and disease.

Switching to a raw food diet nourishes the body in a much more natural way. Vitamins, minerals and enzymes are preserved and glycotoxins caused by high temperatures are kept to a minimum. Eliminating gluten and dairy, two of the main offending proteins, also contributes to fighting inflammation and disease. Many people who have made the switch saw their lives being transformed. Chronic painful conditions such as arthritis and fibromyalgia were even reversed for several of them due to the reduction of inflammation throughout the body.

Creating delicious raw, gluten- and dairy-free dishes sounds scarier than it actually is. Just taking the time to learn how to perfect this art could literally transform your life. Many raw food advocates prefer a vegan approach, since raw animal products are often unsafe for consumption. Whether you decide to include meat and eggs or not is usually a personal choice. If you opt for an omnivore raw food diet, make sure you buy from local, organic producers and consume the meat as fresh as possible.

This book will guide you on your journey to discovering a much healthier way of eating. You'll find many recipes that are not only delicious but easy to make. You can purée, juice, dehydrate or dry raw foods to preserve their natural enzymes and healing properties. You can even gently heat them, as long as the temperature never reaches above the generally accepted threshold of 110-120 degrees Farenheit.

Foods to Avoid

You will want to avoid:

- Gluten-containing grains: rye, barley and wheat, along with kamut, spelt, triticale and other forms of wheat. More often than not, oats are contaminated with wheat during harvesting and processing and should also be avoided. In fact, all grains should be limited or eliminated. However, you can consume small amounts of millet, quinoa and buckwheat by sprouting them, improving their digestibility when consumed in their raw form.

- All foods cooked above 110-120 degrees Farenheit. In fact, the lower the better. Avoid anything that has been heated above this threshold as well, such as pasteurized honey and tea made with boiling water.

- Store-bought meat and eggs: these are at high risk of contamination and should preferably never be consumed raw. Ground steak from one package contains meat from an astonishing 2000 animals in some cases, effectively increasing the possibility of bacterial contamination. Instead, seek out local farmers who sell fresh and preferably organic products. Another option is to go raw vegan.

- All dairy: this includes butter, ice cream, milk, cheese, whey, milk by-products, yogurt and more. Most people are able to tolerate clarified butter, or ghee, with no adverse effects. Ghee has been separated to remove the milk solids (protein and sugar) so that only milk fat remains. Fat does not generally cause intolerances in most people, as opposed to proteins and sugars.

- Processed foods are to be avoided. Few of them can actually fit in the "raw, gluten- and dairy-free" category. Furthermore, processed food is generally filled with preservatives, added sugar and other toxic food additives. If you're looking to be healthier, avoiding processed foods is one of the first moves you can make.

Breakfast Recipes

Choco-cado Smoothie

Prep Time: 10 minutes*

Servings: 1

INGREDIENTS

1/2 cup raw almonds

1 avocado

2 - 4 tablespoons raw cocoa powder

1/4 - 1/2 cup dried pitted dates

Water

INSTRUCTIONS

1. *Soak almonds in enough water to cover at least 6 hours, or overnight. Drain and rinse. Soak dates in enough water to cover at least 6 hours, or overnight. Drain.

2. Add soaked almonds to high-speed blender with 1 1/2 - 2 cups water. Process until well blended and almost smooth, about 1- 2 minutes.

3. Strain mixture through nut milk bag, cheesecloth or strainer back into blender.

4. Cut avocado in half and remove pit. Scoop flesh into blender with soaked dates and cocoa powder.

5. Process until smooth, about 1 minute,.

6. Pour into serving glass and serve immediately.

Pineapple Coconut Smoothie

Prep Time: 10 minutes*

Servings: 1

INSTRUCTIONS

1 fresh coconut (or 1/2 cup flaked coconut)

1/2 cup pineapple chunks (fresh or frozen)

1 cup ice (crushed preferably)

Water

DIRECTIONS

1. *Soak flaked coconut in 1 1/2 cups water in refrigerator overnight, if using.
2. Add soaked coconut and soaking liquid to high-speed blender. Or remove flesh from fresh coconut and add to high-speed blender with 1 1/2 cups water. Process until well blended and fairly smooth, about 1 - 2 minutes.
3. Strain mixture through nut milk bag, cheesecloth or strainer back into blender.
4. Reserve pulp and set aside to dry and dehydrate, then use as coconut flour.
5. Cut pineapple flesh from peel, then chop. Add to blender with ice. Process until smooth, about 1 - 2 minutes.
6. Pour into serving glass and serve immediately.

Ginger Orange Burst

Prep Time: 5 minutes

Servings: 1

INGREDIENTS

3 oranges

1/2 grapefruit

3 large carrots

1 inch piece fresh ginger

Water (optional)

INSTRUCTIONS

1. Peel orange , grapefruit and ginger. Separate citrus segments and add to high-speed blender with carrots and ginger. Process until smooth, about 2 minutes. Add enough water to reach desired consistency.
2. Or peel and cut orange and grapefruit in half, and run through juicer with carrots and ginger.
3. Or cut orange and grapefruit in half and juice with citrus juicer. Then run carrots and ginger through juicer and add to citrus juice.
4. Pour into serving glass and serve immediately.

Berry Breakfast Parfait

Prep Time: 10 minutes*

Servings: 2

INGREDIENTS

1/2 cup raw walnuts

1/2 cup raw almonds

1/4 cup raw pumpkin seeds

1/4 cup raw sunflower seeds

1/4 cup raw flax seeds

1 cup blueberries

1 cup raspberries

Vanilla Cream

1 cup raw cashews

2 tablespoons raw honey (or dried pitted dates)

1/2 teaspoon vanilla

1/8 teaspoon Celtic sea salt

Water

INSTRUCTIONS

1. *Soak cashews and dates (if using) in enough water to cover at least 6 hours, or overnight in refrigerator. Drain and set aside.

2. Add walnuts, almonds, pumpkin, sunflower and flax seeds to food processor or high-speed blender. Pulse to coarsely chop. Set aside.

3. For *Vanilla Cream*, add soaked cashews, honey or dates, vanilla and salt to clean food processor or high-speed blender. Process

until smooth, about 1 - 2 minutes. Add enough water or nut milk to reach desired consistency.

4. Spoon layer of fruit into serving dish. Top with chopped nuts. Spoon on layer of *Vanilla Cream*. Add second layer of chopped nuts. Top with layer of fruit.

5. Serve immediately. Or refrigerate 20 minutes and serve chilled.

Mexican Chocolate Chia Pudding

Prep Time: 10 minutes*

Servings: 2

INGREDIENTS

2 coconuts (or 1 cup flaked coconut)

6 dried pitted dates

3 tablespoons whole chia seeds

2 tablespoons cocoa powder

1/2 teaspoon vanilla

1/2 teaspoon ground black pepper

Pinch cayenne pepper

Pinch chili powder

Pinch smoked paprika

Water

INSTRUCTIONS

1. *Soak flaked coconut in 2 cups water overnight in refrigerator, if using. Soak dates in enough water to cover at least 4 hours, or overnight in refrigerator. Drain dates.

2. Add soaked coconut and soaking liquid to high-speed blender. Or remove flesh from fresh coconuts and add to high-speed blender with 2 cups water. Process until well blended and fairly smooth, about 1 - 2 minutes.

3. Strain mixture through nut milk bag, cheesecloth or strainer back into blender.

4. Reserve pulp and set aside to dry and dehydrate, then use as coconut flour.
5. Add dates, cocoa, vanilla and spices to blender. Process until smooth, about 1 minute.
6. Pour mixture into serving dish and stir in chia seeds. Set aside to thicken, about 1 minute.
7. Serve immediately. Or refrigerate 20 minutes and serve chilled.

Awesome Strawberry Chia Pudding

Prep Time: 10 minutes*

Servings: 2

INGREDIENTS

2 coconuts (or 1 cup flaked coconut)

2 - 4 tablespoons raw honey (or dried pitted dates)

1/4 cup tablespoons whole chia seeds

1 cup strawberries (fresh or frozen and thawed, chopped)

1/2 teaspoon vanilla

Water

INSTRUCTIONS

1. *Soak flaked coconut in 2 cups water overnight in refrigerator, if using. Soak dates in enough water to cover at least 4 hours, or overnight in refrigerator, if using. Drain dates.
2. Add soaked coconut and soaking liquid to high-speed blender. Or remove flesh from fresh coconuts and add to high-speed blender with 2 cups water. Process until well blended and fairly smooth, about 1 - 2 minutes.
3. Strain mixture through nut milk bag, cheesecloth or strainer back into blender.
4. Reserve pulp and set aside to dry and dehydrate, then use as coconut flour.
5. Remove stems from strawberries, then cut in half. Add to blender with honey or dates, and vanilla. Process until smooth, about 1 minute.

6. Pour mixture into serving dish and stir in chia seeds. Set aside to thicken, about 1 minute.

7. Serve immediately. Or refrigerate 20 minutes and serve chilled.

Wholesome Coconut Banana Porridge

Prep Time: 10 minutes

Servings: 2

INGREDIENTS

1 coconut (1/2 cup flaked coconut)

3/4 cup raw nuts (any combination of cashews, almonds, brazil nuts, acorns, macadamia nuts, etc.)

2 overripe bananas

2 teaspoons ground cinnamon

1/4 teaspoon vanilla

1/4 teaspoon Celtic sea salt

Water

INSTRUCTIONS

1. * Soak nuts in enough water to cover for at least 6 hours, or overnight in refrigerator. Drain and rinse, then set aside. Soak flaked coconut in 2 cups water in refrigerator overnight, if using.

2. Add soaked coconut and soaking liquid to high-speed blender. Or remove flesh from fresh coconut and add to high-speed blender with 2 cups water. Process until well blended and fairly smooth, about 1 - 2 minutes.

3. Strain mixture through nut milk bag, cheesecloth or strainer back into blender or food processor.

4. Reserve pulp and set aside to dry and dehydrate, then use as coconut flour.

5. Peel bananas and add to processor with vanilla, salt and 1 teaspoon cinnamon. Process until thick and mostly smooth, about 1 minute.
6. Transfer to serving dish and serve immediately.

Sweet Cocoa Chia Bars

Prep Time: 25 minutes

Servings: 6

INGREDIENTS

1 cup dried pitted dates

3/4 cup raw nuts (any combination of cashews, almonds, brazil nuts, acorns, macadamia nuts, etc.)

2 tablespoon raw cocoa powder

2 tablespoons chia seeds

1/2 teaspoon ground cinnamon

1/2 teaspoon vanilla

Pinch ground black pepper

Pinch Celtic sea salt

1/3 cup warm water

INSTRUCTIONS

1. Soak dates in warm water 5 - 10 minutes, then drain.
2. Line loaf pan with parchment paper.
3. Add nuts to food processor or high-speed blender with soaked dates, cocoa, cinnamon, vanilla, salt and pepper. Process for about 1 minute, until dates and nuts break down and mixture sticks together when pressed.
4. Transfer mixture to small mixing bowl and add chia seeds. Mix with large spoon until well combined, about 1 minute.
5. Transfer mixture to prepared loaf pan and press firmly into bottom with hands or spatula.

6. Place in refrigerator and chill for 10 minutes. Then remove and cut into 6 bars.

7. Serve immediately. Or store in refrigerator up to 2 weeks.

Apricot Mango Breakfast Bars

Prep Time: 25 minutes

Servings: 6

INGREDIENTS

3/4 cup dried apricots

3/4 cup dried mango slices

1 1/4 cup raw nuts (any combination of cashews, almonds, brazil nuts, acorns, macadamia nuts, etc.)

1/2 teaspoon ground ginger

1/4 teaspoon vanilla

1/3 cup warm water

1 lemon

INSTRUCTIONS

1. Juice lemon and add to bowl with warm water and fruit. Soak 5 - 10 minutes, then drain.
2. Line loaf pan with parchment paper.
3. Add nuts to food processor or high-speed blender with soaked fruit, ginger and vanilla. Process for about 1 minute, until fruit and nuts break down and mixture sticks together when pressed.
4. Transfer mixture to prepared loaf pan and press firmly into bottom with hands or spatula.
5. Place in refrigerator and chill for 10 minutes. Then remove and cut into 6 bars.
6. Serve immediately. Or store in refrigerator up to 2 weeks.

Carrot Cranberry Crunch Salad

Prep Time: 5 minutes

Servings: 1

INSTRUCTIONS

2 large carrots

3 tablespoon dried cranberries

1/4 cup raw almonds

1/2 small orange (or tangerine)

1/2 piece fresh ginger

1/2 teaspoon ground ginger

DIRECTIONS

1. Add carrots to food processor with shredding attachment and process, or grate with grater. Add to medium mixing bowl with cranberries and ground ginger.

2. Add almonds to food processor and pulse to coarsely chop. Or add to paper or plastic kitchen bag and pound with heavy rolling pin to crush. Peel ginger and dice or finely grate. Zest *then* juice orange. Add to carrot mixture and toss to combine.

3. Transfer to serving dish and serve immediately. Or refrigerate 20 minutes and serve chilled.

Hearty Apple Almond Salad

Prep Time: 5 minutes

Servings: 1

INSTRUCTIONS

1 apple

1 small banana

1/4 cup blueberries

1/4 cup raw almonds

2 dried pitted dates

2 tablespoons pomegranate seeds (or dried goji or noni berries)

1/4 teaspoon ground cinnamon

INGREDIENTS

1. Core and dice apple. Peel and dice banana. Add to serving dish and mix to combine. Top with blueberries.
2. Chop almonds and dates. Or add to food processor and pulse to coarsely grind.
3. Top fruit with chopped nuts and dates. Sprinkle with pomegranate seeds and cinnamon and serve immediately.

Very Berry Morning Mix

Prep Time: 10 minutes

Servings: 1

INSTRUCTIONS

1 nectarine

1/2 cup strawberries

1/4 cup blackberries

1/4 cup blueberry

1/4 cup cherries

1/4 cup raw nuts (cashews, almonds, brazil nuts, acorns, macadamia, etc.)

1/2 inch piece fresh ginger

Small sprig fresh mint

INGREDIENTS

1. Cut nectarine in half and remove pit. Dice and add to small mixing bowl. Remove stems from strawberries and quarter. Pit cherries. Add to bowl with blackberries and blueberries.

2. Peel ginger and mince or finely grate. Chiffon mint leaves. Add to bowl and toss to combine. Transfer to serving dish.

3. Add nuts to food processor and pulse to coarsely chop. Or add to paper or plastic kitchen bag and pound with heavy rolling pin to crush.

4. Sprinkle on nuts and serve immediately. Or refrigerate 20 minutes and serve chilled.

Sweet Citrus Salad with Coconut Cream

Prep Time: 10 minutes

Servings: 1

INSTRUCTIONS

1 fresh coconut (or 1/2 cup flaked coconut)

1/4 - 1/3 cup dried pitted dates (or raw honey)

1 blood orange

1 tangerine (or navel orange or clementine)

1/2 grapefruit (ruby red, pink or white)

1/2 lime

1 tablespoon sunflower seeds (optional)

Water

INGREDIENTS

1. *Soak flaked coconut in 1 cup water overnight in refrigerator, if using. Soak dates in enough water to cover overnight in refrigerator. Drain.

2. Add soaked coconut and soaking liquid to high-speed blender. Or remove flesh from fresh coconut and add to high-speed blender with 3/4 cup water. Process until thick and fairly smooth, about 1 - 2 minutes.

3. Strain mixture through nut milk bag, cheesecloth or strainer back into blender or to food processor.

4. Reserve pulp and set aside to dry and dehydrate, then use as coconut flour.

5. Add soaked dates or honey to processor and process until smooth. Set aside.
6. Peel all citrus and cut into segments. Add to serving dish. Top with sweet coconut cream. Sprinkle on sunflower seeds (optional).
7. Serve immediately. Or refrigerate 20 minutes and serve chilled.

Peaches and Spiced Almonds

Prep Time: 5 minutes

Servings: 1

INGREDIENTS

2 ripe peaches (or nectarines)

4 dried pitted dates

1/3 cup raw almonds

1/4 teaspoon ground cinnamon

1/4 teaspoon ground ginger

1/8 teaspoon vanilla

1/8 teaspoon ground white pepper (or ground black pepper)

INSTRUCTIONS

1. Add dates, almonds vanilla and spices to food processor or high-speed blender. Pulse to coarsely grind, about 1 minute.
2. Cut peaches in half and remove pits. Dice peaches and transfer to serving dish.
3. Sprinkle on almond mixture and serve immediately.

Cream of Cashew Cereal

Prep Time: 5 minutes*

Servings: 1

INGREDIENTS

1 1/2 cups raw cashews

1 banana

1/4 cup blueberries

1 tablespoon raw honey (or 2 pitted dates)

1 tablespoon lemon juice

1/4 teaspoon vanilla

1/4 teaspoon Celtic sea salt

Water

INSTRUCTIONS

1. *Soak cashews and dates (if using) in enough water to cover overnight in refrigerator. Drain.

2. Peel banana. Add to food processor or high-speed blender with soaked cashews, dates or honey, lemon juice, vanilla and salt. Process until thick and fairly smooth, about 1 - 2 minutes. Add enough water to reach desired consistency.

3. Transfer to serving dish and top with blueberries. Serve immediately.

No-Oat Granola Bowl

Prep Time: 10 minutes*

Servings: 1

INGREDIENTS

3/4 cup raw almonds

1/3 cups raw walnuts

1/3 cups cashews

1/4 cup raw pumpkin seeds

1/4 cup shredded or flaked coconut

2 tablespoon dried cranberries

1/3 cup dried pitted dates

1/4 tablespoon vanilla

1/4 tablespoon cinnamon

1/4 teaspoon ground ginger

1/2 teaspoon Celtic sea salt

Water

INSTRUCTIONS

1. *Separately oak 1/4 cup almonds in enough water to cover at least 6 hours, or overnight. Drain and rinse. Soak 1/4 cupdates in enough water to cover at least 6 hours, or overnight. Drain.

2. Add soaked almonds to high-speed blender with 2/3 - 3/4 cup water. Process until well blended and almost smooth, about 1- 2 minutes.

3. Strain mixture through nut milk bag, cheesecloth or strainer back into blender.

4. Add soaked dates to blender with vanilla, salt and ginger. Process until smooth, about 1 minutes. Add to medium mixing bowl.

5. Chop remaining almonds, walnuts and dates by hand. Or add to clean food processor or high-speed blender and pulse to roughly chop. Add to bowl with pumpkin seeds, flaked coconut, cranberries and cinnamon. Mix to combine.

6. Transfer to serving dish and serve immediately. Or refrigerate 20 minutes and serve chilled.

Nutty Oatmeal Bowl

Prep Time: 5 minutes*

Servings: 2

INGREDIENTS

2 cage free eggs (optional)

1/2 apple

1/4 cup flaked or shredded coconut

1/4 - 1/3 cup dried pitted dates

1/3 cup raw walnuts

1/3 cup raw almonds

2 tablespoons coconut oil (or coconut butter or cacao butter)

2 tablespoons flax seed (or chia seed)

2 tablespoons raisins

2 tablespoons dried goji berries (optional)

1 teaspoon ground cinnamon

Pinch Celtic sea salt

Water

INSTRUCTIONS

1. *Soak walnuts and almonds in enough water to cover for at least 6
   hours, or overnight in refrigerator. Drain and rinse, then set aside.
   Soak dates in enough water to cover for at least 6 hours, or
   overnight in refrigerator. Drain and set aside. Soak flaked coconut
   in 1 cup water overnight in refrigerator.

2. Add flax or chia to food processor or high-speed blender and process until finely ground. Add coconut oil and process until thick paste forms.

3. Add dates, nuts, eggs, cinnamon, salt, soaked coconut and soaking liquid to processor. Process until thick mixture forms, about 1 - 2 minutes. Transfer to serving dish.

4. Core and dice apple. Top with dices apple, raisins and goji berries (optional).

5. Serve immediately.

Turkey Jerky Bacon

Prep Time: 10 minutes*

Dehydrating Time: 4 - 8 hours

Servings: 4

INGREDIENTS

4 oz organic turkey (dark meat)

2 tablespoons coconut aminos (or liquid aminos)

2 tablespoons tamari (or liquid aminos or coconut aminos)

1 tablespoon lemon juice (or raw apple cider vinegar)

1 tablespoons Celtic sea salt

1/2 teaspoon garlic powder

1/2 teaspoon onion powder

1/2 teaspoon smoked paprika

Pinch cayenne pepper

INSTRUCTIONS

1. Prepare two sheet parchment. Lay one on cutting board.

2. Cut turkey into 1/4 inch strips and lay in single layer on parchment. Pound with tenderizing side of kitchen mallet. Cover turkey with second parchment sheet, then pound with flat side of tenderizing mallet to 1/8 inch thickness.

3. *Place turkey strips in medium mixing bowl or shallow dish. Add coconut aminos, tamari, lemon juice, salt and spices. Mix well to coat. Cover and place in refrigerator for 8 hours, or overnight.

4. Remove turkey from refrigerator and lay in single layer on dehydrator trays. Place trays in dehydrator and set to 120 degrees F for 4 - 8 hours.

5. After 4 hours dehydrating time, remove trays from dehydrator and test turkey by bending. If it cracks, remove and serve immediately. Or store in airtight container.

6. If still flexible, place back in dehydrator and continue dehydrating up to 4 hours, or until desired texture is achieved.

Crêpes with Cashew Lemon Curd

Prep Time: 15 minutes*

Dehydrating Time: 7 - 10 hours

Servings: 2

INGREDIENTS

Crêpes

1 young coconut (plus coconut water)

1/2 orange

1/2 cup flax seeds

1 tablespoon raw honey (or dried pitted dates)

1 teaspoon ground cinnamon

Lemon Curd

1/3 cup raw cashews

1/4 cup coconut butter(or cacao butter)

2 lemons (1/4 cup juice)

2 - 4 tablespoons raw honey

Pinch Celtic sea salt

Pinch of turmeric (optional)

Water

INSTRUCTIONS

1. For *Crêpes*, add flax to food processor or high-speed blender. Process until finely ground, up to 5 minutes.

2. Remove flesh and water from young coconut. Peel orange and cut into segments. Add to processor with honey and cinnamon. Process until thick and smooth, about 1 - 2 minutes.

3. Place parchment paper or dehydrator sheets on dehydrator trays.

4. Spread batter on prepared sheets. Place trays in dehydrator and set to 115 degrees F for 6 - 8 hours.

5. Remove trays from dehydrator. Remove *Crêpes* from parchment or dehydrator liners, flip, and place directly on dehydrator tray. Place trays back in dehydrator and continue dehydrating 1 - 2 hours, until surface is dry but *Crêpe* is still pliable.

6. Remove from dehydrator and cut into desired shape and size. Set aside.

7. *For *Lemon Curd*, soak cashews in enough water to cover for at least 6 hours, or overnight in refrigerator. Drain and rinse.

8. Zest 1 lemon, then juice lemons into food processor or high-speed blender. Add coconut butter, honey, salt and turmeric, for color (optional).Process until smooth, about 1 - 2 minutes. Add enough water to reach desired consistency.

9. Lay *Crêpes* flat and top with line of *Lemon Curd* down center. Roll up *Crêpes* and transfer to serving dish. Serve immediately.

Lox and Avocado Crêpes

Prep Time: 10 minutes

Dehydrating Time: 7 - 10 hours

Servings: 2

INGREDIENTS

4 - 6 oz smoked salmon

1 ripe avocado

1/2 lemon

1 sprig fresh dill

1 teaspoon sesame seeds (black or white)

Crêpes

1 young coconut (plus coconut water)

1/3 cup raw sunflower seeds

1/2 cup flax seeds

1/2 white ground pepper (or 1/4 teaspoon ground black pepper)

1/2 teaspoon Celtic sea salt

Water

INSTRUCTIONS

1. For *Crêpes*, add flax to food processor or high-speed blender. Process until finely ground, up to 5 minutes. Add sunflower seeds and process until finely ground, about 1 minute.

2. Remove flesh and water from young coconut. Add to processor with salt and pepper. Process until smooth batter forms, about 1 - 2 minutes. Add enough water to reach desired consistency.

3. Place parchment paper or dehydrator sheets on dehydrator trays.

4. Spread batter on prepared sheets. Place trays in dehydrator and set to 115 degrees F for 6 - 8 hours.

5. Remove trays from dehydrator. Remove *Crêpes* from parchment or dehydrator liners, flip, and place directly on dehydrator tray. Place trays back in dehydrator and continue dehydrating 1 - 2 hours, until surface is dry but *Crêpe* is still pliable.

6. Remove from dehydrator and cut into desired shape and size. Set aside.

7. Finely chop fresh dill. Cut avocado in half and remove pit. Slice flesh in peel.

8. Lay *Crêpes* flat and top with line of smoked salmon down center. Scoop portion of sliced avocado over smoked salmon. Sprinkle on chopped dill. Roll up *Crêpes* and transfer to serving dish.

9. Top *Crêpes* with squeeze of lemon juice and sprinkle on sesame seeds. Serve immediately.

Bananarama Pancake Stack

Prep Time: 15 minutes

Dehydrating Time: 8 - 9 hours

Servings: 2

INGREDIENTS

Banana Pancakes

2 overripe bananas

1/2 cup raw cashews (or 1/4 cup raw cashew butter)

1/4 cup flax seed

1 teaspoon ground cinnamon

1/2 teaspoon vanilla

1/2 teaspoon cardamom (optional)

Water

Topping

1 ripe banana

1/4 teaspoon ground cinnamon

1 tablespoon raw honey (or date butter)

INSTRUCTIONS

1. For *Banana Pancakes*, add flax to food processor or high-speed blender. Process until finely ground, about 2 minutes.
2. Add cashews to processor, if using. Process until smooth, up to 5 minutes.

3. Or add cashew butter to processor with bananas, cinnamon, vanilla and cardamom (optional). Process until smooth batter forms, about 1 - 2 minutes. Add enough water to reach desired consistency.

4. Place parchment paper or dehydrator sheets on dehydrator trays.

5. Use spoon to spread batter on prepared sheets in 2 x 2 inch circles 1/4 inch thick. Place trays in dehydrator and set to 110 degrees F for 6 hours.

6. Remove trays from dehydrator. Flip *Banana Pancakes* and place trays back in dehydrator. Continue dehydrating 2 - 3 hours, until surface is dry but *Banana Pancakes* are still moist and pliable.

7. For *Topping*, peel banana and slice. Add to small mixing bowl with cinnamon and honey or date butter. Toss to coat.

8. Remove *Banana Pancakes* from dehydrator and transfer to serving dish. Top with spiced banana *Topping* and serve immediately.

Coconut Pancakes and Berry Jam

Prep Time: 15 minutes*

Dehydrating Time: 8 - 9 hours

Servings: 2

INGREDIENTS

Pancakes

1 young coconut (plus coconut water)

1/2 cup raw cashews (or 1/4 cup raw cashew butter)

1/4 cup flax seed

1/4 teaspoon ground cinnamon

1/2 teaspoon vanilla

Water

Berry Jam

1 orange

1/4 cup dried raspberries

1/4 cup dried cherries

1/4 cup dried strawberries

 Water

INSTRUCTIONS

1. *Soak dried fruit in enough water to cover at least 4 hours, or overnight in refrigerator. Drain and reserve soaking liquid. Set aside.

2. For *Pancakes*, add flax to food processor or high-speed blender. Process until finely ground, about 2 minutes.

3. Add cashews to processor, if using. Process until smooth, up to 5 minutes. Or use prepared cashew butter.

4. Remove flesh and water from young coconut add and add to processor with cashew butter, cinnamon and vanilla cardamom. Process until smooth batter forms, about 1 - 2 minutes. Add enough water to reach desired consistency.

5. Place parchment paper or dehydrator sheets on dehydrator trays.

6. Use spoon to spread batter on prepared sheets in 2 x 2 inch circles 1/4 inch thick. Place trays in dehydrator and set to 110 degrees F for 6 hours.

7. Remove trays from dehydrator. Flip *Pancakes* and place trays back in dehydrator. Continue dehydrating 2 - 3 hours, until surface is dry but *Pancakes* are still moist and pliable.

8. For *Berry Jam*, zest *then* juice orange into clean food processor or high-speed blender. Add soaked fruit and process until mostly smooth, about 1 minute. Add enough soaking liquid and/or water to reach desired consistency and sweetness.

9. Remove *Pancakes* from dehydrator and transfer to serving dish. Top with *Berry Jam* and serve immediately.

Superfood Breakfast Brownies

Prep Time: 10 minutes

Servings: 2

INGREDIENTS

1 cup dried pitted dates

1/2 cup cashews

1/2 cup sunflower seeds

1/4 cup hulled hemp seeds (or chia or flax seeds)

1/4 cup shredded or flaked coconut

1/4 cup raw cocoa powder

2 tablespoons coconut oil (or coconut butter or cacao butter)

1 teaspoon vanilla

1/4 teaspoon Celtic sea salt

Pinch ground black pepper.

1/4 cup raw cacao nibs (or dried goji berries, noni berries, pomegranates seeds, or any combination)

INSTRUCTIONS

1. Add hemp, chia or flax seeds sunflower seeds to food processor or high-speed blender. Process until finely ground, about 2 minutes. Add sunflower seeds and process until finely ground, about 1 minute. Add cashews and process until finely ground, about 1 minute.

2. Add dates in batches and continue processing until mixture is well ground and sticks together.

3. Add coconut, cocoa , coconut oil, vanilla, salt and pepper. Process about 30 seconds to incorporate.

4. Transfer to medium mixing bowl and add cacao nibs, dried berries or pomegranate seeds. Mix to combine.

5. Transfer mixture to lined loaf pan and press into bottom with hands or spatula. Slice and serve. Or refrigerate 20 minutes to firm, then slice and serve.

Coconut Cake Breakfast Plate

Prep Time: 10 minutes*

Servings: 2

INGREDIENTS

Coconut Breakfast Cake

1 fresh coconut (or 1/2 cup flaked or shredded coconut)

1/2 cup ground flax seed (or chia seed)

1/4 cup raw honey (or 1/3 cup dried pitted dates)

2 tablespoons coconut oil (or coconut butter or cacao butter)

1/2 teaspoon ground cinnamon

1/4 teaspoon Celtic sea salt

Water

Apricot Jam

1 cup dried apricots

2 tablespoons lemon juice

1/4 inch piece fresh ginger (or 1/2 teaspoon ground ginger)

Water

INSTRUCTIONS

1. *For *Coconut Breakfast Cakes*, soak flaked coconut and in 1 cup water overnight in refrigerator, if using. Soak dates in enough water to cover overnight in refrigerator, if using. Drain.

2. Add soaked coconut and soaking liquid to high-speed blender. Or remove flesh from fresh coconut and add to high-speed blender with 1 cup water, ground flax or chia, soaked dates or honey,

coconut oil, salt and cinnamon. Pulse to coarsely grind, until mixture sticks together.

3. Form mixture into 6 balls and flatten into cakes. Or mold in lined muffin tins. Set aside.

4. For *Apricot Jam*, peel ginger and add to clean food processor or high-speed blender with apricots and lemon juice. Process until smooth, about 1 minute. Add enough water to reach desired consistency.

5. Transfer *Coconut Breakfast Cakes* to serving dish. Top with *Apricot Jam* and serve immediately. Or refrigerate 20 minutes and serve chilled.

Carrot Biscuits with Sweet Tahini

Prep Time: 20 minutes

Servings: 6

INGREDIENTS

Carrot Biscuit

3 large carrots (1 1/2 cups shredded)

1/3 - 1/2 cup dried pitted dates

1/2 cup raw walnuts

1/3 cup shredded or flaked coconut

1/4 cup raisins (optional)

1/2 teaspoon ground cinnamon

1/2 teaspoon ground ginger

1/4 teaspoon Celtic sea salt

Pinch ground nutmeg

Pinch ground black pepper

Sweet Tahini

1 cup raw sesame seeds (or 1/2 cup raw tahini)

1/4 cup raw pitted dates (or 3 tablespoon raw honey)

1 tablespoon lemon juice

INSTRUCTIONS

1. For *Carrot Biscuit*, add carrots, dates, walnuts, coconut, salt and spices to food processor or high-speed blender. Pulse to coarsely grind, until mixture sticks together.
2. Transfer to small mixing bowl and stir in raisins (optional).

3. Form mixture into 6 balls and flatten into biscuits. Or mold in lined muffin tins. Set aside.

4. For *Sweet Tahini*, add raw sesame seeds to clean food processor or high-speed blender and process until smooth, up to 5 minutes. Add dates or honey and lemon juice.

5. Or add prepared tahini to clean food processor or high-speed blender with dates or raw honey and lemon juice. Process until smooth, about 1 - 2 minutes.

6. Transfer *Carrot Biscuits* to serving dish. Top with *Sweet Tahini* and serve immediately. Or refrigerate 20 minutes and serve chilled.

Lunch Recipes

Mexican Tomato Soup

Prep Time: 35 minutes

Servings: 2

INGREDIENTS

Shrimp

10 - 12 large shrimp

1 - 1 1/2 cups lemon juice (about 8 lemons)

1/2 jalapeño pepper

Gazpacho

2 cups tomato juice (about 4 large tomatoes)

2 plum tomatoes

1/2 red bell pepper

1/2 red onion

1/2 cucumber

Small bunch fresh cilantro

2 garlic cloves

2 tablespoons raw apple cider vinegar(optional)

2 tablespoons raw oil (coconut, walnut, almond, sesame, etc.) (optional)

1 teaspoon ground black pepper

1 teaspoon Celtic sea salt

INSTRUCTIONS

1. For *Shrimp*, Peel, devein and remove tails from shrimp. Mince jalapeño and juice lemons. Add to small bowl and mix. Shrimp

should be completely covered in lemon juice. Place in refrigerator for 30 minutes, or until shrimp are opaque.

2. For Gazpacho, juice large tomatoes in juicer. Or add to food processor or high-speed blender and process, then strain into medium mixing bowl.

3. Peel cucumber and seed. Seed plum tomatoes. Seed, stem and vein bell peppers. Peel onion and garlic. Dice veggies and onion, and mince garlic. Add to tomato juice.

4. Add salt, pepper, vinegar and oil (optional). Mix well, then place in refrigerator.

5. Chop cilantro and set aside.

6. Remove shrimp from refrigerator and drain lemon juice and jalapeños. Rinse if desired.

7. Mix shrimp into tomato mixture. Pour into serving bowls and top with chopped cilantro. Serve chilled.

Carrot Ginger Soup

Prep Time: 10 minutes

Servings: 2

INGREDIENTS

3 large carrots

1/2 cup fresh young coconut meat (about 1/2 young coconut)

1/4 cup raw pine nuts (or raw cashews)

1/2 - 1 inch piece fresh ginger

2 sprigs fresh cilantro

1 tablespoon coconut aminos (or raw apple cider vinegar)

1/2 teaspoon fresh cracked black pepper

Water (or coconut milk)

INSTRUCTIONS

1. Remove cilantro leaves from stems and add to highs-speed blender. Juice ginger, or peel and finely grate. Add to blender with pine nuts, coconut, and coconut aminos.

2. Juice carrots, or add to food processor or high-speed blender and process until smooth, about 2 minutes. Add enough water or coconut milk to reach desired consistency.

3. Pour into serving bowls and top with fresh cracked black pepper. Serve immediately.

Tomato Basil Soup

Prep Time: 10 minutes

Servings: 2

INGREDIENTS

5 - 6 plum tomatoes

2 sundried tomatoes

1 clove garlic

1/4 cup raw cashews

1 sprig fresh basil (or 1/2 teaspoon dried basil)

1 sprig fresh oregano (or 1/2 teaspoon dried oregano)

1/4 teaspoon ground white pepper (or ground black pepper)

1/2 teaspoon Celtic sea salt

Water

INSTRUCTIONS

1. Juice plum tomatoes. Or add to food processor or high-speed blender and process. Add enough water to reach desired consistency, if necessary. Then strain.
2. Peel garlic, and remove basil and oregano leaves from stems, if using. Add basil and oregano to food processor or high-speed blender with tomato juice, sundried tomatoes, cashews, salt and pepper. Process until smooth, about 2 minutes.
3. Pour into serving bowls and serve immediately.

Texas Chili

Prep Time: 10 minutes*

Servings: 2

INGREDIENTS

5 - 6 plum tomatoes

1/2 teaspoon dried cumin

1/4 teaspoon chili powder

1/4 teaspoon onion powder

1/4 teaspoon garlic powder

1 teaspoon fresh oregano leaves (or 1/4 teaspoon dried oregano)

1/2 teaspoon ground black pepper

1/4 teaspoon cayenne pepper or red pepper flakes (optional)

1 teaspoon Celtic sea salt

1 teaspoon chia seed (or flax seed)

1/2 cup raw cashews

Water

INSTRUCTIONS

1. *Soak raw cashews in enough water to cover overnight in refrigerator. Drain and rinse. Set aside.
2. Grind chia or flax in food processor or high-speed blender. Set aside.
3. Juice tomatoes. Or add to food processor or high-speed blender and process. Add enough water to reach desired consistency, if necessary. Then strain.

4. Add tomato juice, ground chia or flax, 1/2 of soaked cashews, salt, pepper and spices to blender. Process until smooth, about 1 - 2 minutes.
5. Stir in remaining soaked cashews.
6. Pour into serving bowls and serve immediately.

Creamy "Cheese" and Broccoli Soup

Prep Time: 10 minutes*

Servings: 2

INGREDIENTS

1 1/2 - 2 cups broccoli florets

1 red bell pepper

1 garlic clove

1/4 cup raw oil (coconut, walnut, almond, sesame, etc.)

1 cup nutritional yeast

1 tablespoon coconut aminos (or tamari)

1 tablespoon onion powder

1/2 teaspoon Celtic sea salt

1/4 teaspoon ground white pepper (or ground black pepper)

2 cups raw cashews

Water

INSTRUCTIONS

1. * Soak raw cashews in enough water to cover at least 2 hours, or overnight in refrigerator. Drain and rinse. Set aside.

2. Chop broccoli florets into pieces and set aside.

3. Seed and vein bell pepper. Peel garlic. Add to food processor or high-speed blender with soaked cashews, nutritional yeast, coconut aminos, salt, pepper and enough water to process until smooth, about 2 - 3 minutes.

4. Pour into serving bowl and top with broccoli. Serve immediately.

Raspberry Almond Salad

Prep Time: 10 minutes

Servings: 1

INGREDIENTS

Salad

2 cups soft lettuce leaves (looseleaf or butterhead varieties)

1/2 cup watercress

2 tablespoons raw almonds (slivered or sliced)

1/4 cup fresh raspberries

Raspberry Vinaigrette

1/4 cup raspberries (fresh or frozen)

2 tablespoons lemon juice (or raw apple cider vinegar)

2 tablespoons raw walnuts (or raw walnut oil, coconut oil, almond oil, etc.)

1 teaspoon sweetener* (optional)

Water

INSTRUCTIONS

1. For *Salad*, rinse, dry and plate lettuce and watercress. Sprinkle almonds and fresh raspberries over greens.

2. For *Raspberry Vinaigrette*, add raspberries, lemon juice, walnuts or oil, and sweetener (optional) to food processor or high-speed blender and process until smooth, about 1 minute. Add enough water to reach desired consistency.

3. Drizzle *Raspberry Vinaigrette* over salad and serve immediately.

stevia, raw honey or dried dates

Caesar Salad

Prep Time: 10 minutes

Servings: 1

INGREDIENTS

2 cups chopped romaine lettuce

Almond Parmesan

1/4 cup raw almonds

1 teaspoon raw apple cider vinegar

1 teaspoon nutritional yeast (optional)

1/4 teaspoon garlic powder

1/4 teaspoon onion powder

1/4 teaspoon dried oregano

1/4 teaspoon Celtic sea salt

Raw Caesar Dressing

2 tablespoons raw cashews (or raw sunflower seeds)

2 tablespoons raw sunflower seeds

1 tablespoon raw pine nuts (or raw sesame seeds or raw tahini)

2 tablespoons lemon juice

1 teaspoon sweetener*

1 garlic clove

3/4 teaspoon coconut aminos (or nutritional yeast)

1/2 teaspoon dried dill (optional)

Cracked or ground black pepper, to taste

Water

INSTRUCTIONS

1. Rinse, dry and plate romaine lettuce.

2. For *Almond Parmesan*, add almonds, vinegar, salt, spices and nutritional yeast (optional) to food processor or high-speed blender. Process until almonds are coarsely ground and resemble ground parmesan cheese. Set aside.

3. For *Raw Caesar Dressing*, peel garlic and add to food processor or high-speed blender with sweetener and lemon juice. Process until smooth. Then add remaining ingredients and process until smooth, about 1 - 2 minutes. Add enough water to reach desired consistency.

4. Drizzle *Raw Caesar Dressing* over salad and sprinkle with *Almond Parmesan*. Serve immediately.

* raw honey or dried dates

Spiced Walnut Autumn Salad

Prep Time: 10 minutes

Servings: 1

INGREDIENTS

Salad

2 cups red lettuce leaves (or other colorful lettuce variety)

1/2 cup arugula

1/2 ripe pear

Spiced Walnuts

1/4 cup walnuts (halves or pieces)

1 tablespoons raw honey (or 1 dried date plus 1 tablespoon water)

1/4 teaspoon ground cinnamon

1/8 teaspoon ground ginger

1/4 teaspoon fresh ground nutmeg

1/8 teaspoon vanilla

1/4 teaspoon ground cardamom (optional)

Orange Vinaigrette

1 orange

2 tablespoons raw apple cider vinegar

2 teaspoons sweetener*

1 teaspoon raw walnut oil (or coconut, almond, sesame oil, etc.)

1 teaspoon raw tahini or sesame seeds (optional)

1 teaspoon ground mustard seeds (or whole mustard seeds)

1/4 teaspoon cracked or ground black pepper

INSTRUCTIONS

1. For *Salad*, rinse, dry and plate lettuce and arugula. Slice pear in half, and remove seeds. Top greens with sliced pears.

2. For *Spiced Walnuts*, process date and water in food processor or high-speed blender until smooth and add to small mixing bowl, if using. Or combine walnuts, spices and raw honey in small mixing bowl. Sprinkle over *Salad*.

3. For *Orange Vinaigrette*, zest and juice orange. Add to food processor or high-speed blender with vinegar, sweetener, spices and tahini (optional) and process until smooth, about 1 minute.

4. Drizzle *Orange Vinaigrette* over salad and serve immediately.

*stevia, raw honey or dried dates

Blueberry Poppy Seed Salad

Prep Time: 10 minutes*

Servings: 1

INGREDIENTS

Salad

2 cups lettuce leaves

1/2 cup dandelion leaves (optional)

2 tablespoons raw almonds (sliced or slivered)

1/4 cup fresh blueberries

Lemon Poppy Seed Dressing

3 tablespoons raw oil (coconut, walnut, almond, sesame, etc.)

2 tablespoons lemon juice

1 tablespoons sweetener*

1/4 teaspoon Celtic sea salt

1 tablespoon poppy seeds

1/4 cup raw cashews

Water

INSTRUCTIONS

1. *Soak cashews in enough water to cover for 30 minutes. Drain and rinse.

2. For *Salad*, rinse, dry and plate lettuce and dandelion leaves (optional). Sprinkle almonds and fresh blueberries over greens.

3. For *Lemon Poppy Seed Dressing*, add soaked cashews, oil, lemon juice, sweetener and salt to food processor or high-speed blender and process until smooth, about 1 - 2 minutes. Stir in poppy seeds.

4. Drizzle *Lemon Poppy Seed Dressing* over salad and serve immediately.

*stevia, raw honey or dried dates

Pecan Apricot Spinach Salad

Prep Time: 10 minutes

Servings: 1

INGREDIENTS

Salad

2 cups spinach leaves

1/2 cup chopped kale leaves

4 - 5 dried apricots

3 tablespoons pecans (halves or pieces)

Honey Mustard Vinaigrette

2 tablespoons raw honey (or 2 dried dates + 2 tablespoons water)

2 tablespoons ground mustard (or mustard seed)

2 tablespoons raw apple cider vinegar

3 tablespoons raw oil (coconut, walnut, almond, sesame, etc.)

3/4 teaspoons Celtic sea salt

INSTRUCTIONS

1. For *Salad*, rinse, dry and plate spinach and kale. Chop dried apricots. Sprinkle apricots and pecans over greens.
2. For *Honey Mustard Vinaigrette*, add honey, mustard, vinegar, oil and salt to food processor or high-speed blender and process until smooth, about 1 minute.
3. Drizzle *Honey Mustard Vinaigrette* over salad and serve immediately.

Smoked Salmon Avocado Salad

Prep Time: 10 minutes

Servings: 1

INGREDIENTS

Salad

2 cups soft lettuce leaves (looseleaf or butterhead varieties)

1/2 cup watercress or dandelion leaves (optional)

2 oz smoked salmon

1/2 avocado

1 sprig fresh dill

1 tablespoon caviar (optional)

Avocado Cream Dressing

1/2 avocado

1 sprig fresh dill

1 tablespoon lemon juice

1/2 teaspoon ground black pepper

1/2 teaspoon Celtic sea salt

1/2 coconut

Water

INSTRUCTIONS

1. For *Salad*, rinse, dry and plate lettuce and watercress or dandelion leaves (optional). Cut avocado in half and remover pit. Dice or slice avocado flesh in peel, then scoop onto greens. Lay smoked salmon over greens.

2. For *Avocado Cream Dressing*, remove coconut flesh from peel and add to food processor or high-speed blender with enough water to reach desired consistency. Process until smooth and creamy, about 1 - 2 minutes. Strain mixture through nut milk bag and place back into blender.

3. Scoop remaining avocado flesh into blender. Add lemon juice, 1 sprig dill, salt and pepper and process until well combined and smooth, about 1 minute.

4. Drizzle *Avocado Cream Dressing* over salad. Mince remaining dill and sprinkle over salad. Dollop caviar over salad (optional).

5. Serve immediately.

*stevia, raw honey or dried dates

Avocado Persimmon Salad

Prep Time: 10 minutes*

Servings: 2

INGREDIENTS

2 persimmons

1 avocado

1 medium cucumber

1/2 sweet onion

2 tablespoons raw oil (coconut, walnut, almond, sesame, etc.)

2 tablespoon lemon juice (or lime juice or raw apple cider vinegar)

1/2 teaspoon cracked or ground black pepper

1/4 teaspoon Celtic sea salt

INSTRUCTIONS

1. Peel and seed cucumber if preferred, then dice. Peel persimmons if preferred, then chop. Peel sweet onions and cut in half. Thinly slice. Add to medium mixing bowl.
2. Cut avocado in half and remove pit. Dice peel in flesh and scoop into bowl.
3. Add oil, lemon juice, salt and pepper. Toss to coat evenly
4. Transfer to serving dishes and serve immediately.
5. *Or refrigerate for 20 minutes and serve chilled.

Sweet Guava Salad

Prep Time: 10 minutes*

Servings: 2

INGREDIENTS

2 ripe guavas

1 personal papaya (1 cup diced papaya flesh)

1 young coconut

1/2 teaspoon ground ginger (or 1/4 inch piece fresh ginger)

2 tablespoons fresh orange juice (about 1/2 orange)

INSTRUCTIONS

1. Dice guavas and add to medium mixing bowl. Peel papaya and cut in half, remove seeds and dice flesh. Remove coconut flesh from shell and dice. Add to bowl.

2. Juice orange into bowl and add ground ginger. Or peel fresh ginger and mince, then add to bowl. Toss to coat fruit evenly.

3. Transfer to serving dishes and serve immediately.

4. *Or refrigerate for 20 minutes and serve chilled.

Cocoa Banana Salad

Prep Time: 5 minutes

Servings: 1

INGREDIENTS

1 banana

2 tablespoons raw almonds

1 tablespoon raw cocoa powder

1 teaspoon raw honey (or coconut cream)

1/4 teaspoon vanilla

1/4 teaspoon cinnamon

1/4 teaspoon smoked paprika (optional)

INSTRUCTIONS

1. Peel banana and chop. Add to small mixing bowl with cocoa powder, honey or coconut cream, almonds, cinnamon, and paprika (optional). Toss to coat evenly.
2. Transfer to serving dish and serve immediately.

Coconut Beet Salad

Prep Time: 10 minutes*

Servings: 1

INGREDIENTS

1 beet

1/2 young coconut

2 tablespoons raw cocoa powder

2 tablespoons coconut cream (or coconut milk)

1/4 teaspoon vanilla

1/4 teaspoon ground black pepper

Pinch Celtic sea salt

INSTRUCTIONS

1. Peel beet and remove coconut flesh from shell. Grate beet and coconut with grater, or add to food processor with shredding attachment and process.
2. Add to medium mixing bowl with cocoa powder, coconut cream, vanilla, salt and pepper. Toss to coat evenly
3. Transfer to serving dish and serve immediately.

Thai Coconut Curry

Prep Time: 20 minutes

Servings: 2

INGREDIENTS

1 tomato

1 carrot

1/2 red pepper

1/2 lemon

1/2 mango

2 cups cauliflower florets

1/2 small onion

1 teaspoon Celtic sea salt

Coconut Curry Sauce

1/2 cup fresh coconut

1/2 lemon

1 lemongrass stem

1 inch piece fresh ginger

1 garlic clove

1 tablespoon fresh curry leaves

Medium bunch fresh parsley

1/2 teaspoon red pepper flakes

1 teaspoon Celtic sea salt

Water

INSTRUCTIONS

1. Seed and chop bell pepper. Seed tomato if preferred, then chop. Dice carrot. Add to medium mixing bowl. Add juice of 1/2 lemon and 1/2 teaspoon salt. Mix and set aside.

2. For *Coconut Curry Sauce*, peel ginger and garlic. Remove coconut flesh from shell and chop. Remove half of parsley from stem. Add to food processor or high-speed blender with lemongrass, lemon juice, curry leaves, salt and red pepper. Process until smooth and creamy, about 1 - 2 minutes. Add enough water to reach desired consistency.

3. Add *Coconut Curry Sauce* to mixing bowl with veggies. Toss to coat and refrigerate at least 10 minutes.

4. Peel onion. Add cauliflower and onion to food processor with shredding attachment and process to "rice." Or mince cauliflower and onion. Add to medium mixing bowl with 1/2 teaspoon salt and mix to combine.

5. Cut mango in half around pit, peel and dice. Chop remaining parsley.

6. Plate "rice" mixture and top with *Coconut Curry Sauce* . Sprinkle mango and parsley over curry. Serve immediately.

Banana Cashew Curry

Prep Time: 10 minutes*

Servings: 2

INGREDIENTS

2 cups cauliflower florets

1 banana

1 teaspoon Celtic sea salt

1/2 cup raw cashews

Water

Cashew Curry Sauce

1/2 cup raw cashews

1/2 red bell pepper

1 small leek

2 teaspoon coconut aminos (or tamari)

Juice of 1/2 lemon

2 teaspoons curry powder

1 teaspoon ground turmeric

1/4 teaspoon cayenne pepper

1/4 teaspoon Celtic sea salt

Water

INSTRUCTIONS

1. *Soak 1/2 cup cashews in enough water to cover over night in refrigerator. Drain and rinse.

2. For *Cashew Curry Sauce*, add cashews to food processor or high-speed blender and process until finely ground.

3. Seed and chop bell pepper. Chop leek. Add to ground cashews with coconut aminos, lemon juice, salt and spices. Process until smooth and creamy, about 1 - 2 minutes. Add enough water to reach desired consistency.

4. Add cauliflower to food processor with shredding attachment and process to "rice." Or mince cauliflower and add to medium mixing bowl with 1/2 teaspoon salt and mix to combine.

5. Peel banana and dice.

6. Plate "rice" mixture and top with diced banana and soaked cashews. Top with *Cashew Curry Sauce*. Serve immediately.

Pesto Tomato Caprese

Prep Time: 5 minutes

Servings: 2

INGREDIENTS

1 large yellow tomato

1 large red tomato

Small bunch fresh basil

Celtic sea salt, to taste

Crack or ground black pepper, to taste

Basil Pesto

2 cups basil leaves (packed)

1/4 cup raw pine nuts

1/2 - 1/3 cup raw oil (coconut, walnut, almond, sesame, etc.)

2 garlic cloves

1/2 lemon (or 1 tablespoon raw apple cider vinegar)

1/4 teaspoon Celtic sea salt

INSTRUCTIONS

1. For *Basil Pesto*, peel garlic and add to food processor or high-speed blender with squeeze of 1/2 lemon. Process until finely chopped. Add pine nuts, basil, oil and salt and process until finely ground, about 1 minute.

2. Slice tomatoes and plate in alternating colors. Sprinkle with salt and pepper. Chiffon basil leaves.

3. Spread *Basil Pesto* over tomato slices and top with fresh basil. Serve immediately.

Cilantro Taco Salad

Prep Time: 10 minutes

Servings: 1

INGREDIENTS

Salad

2 cups lettuce (chopped)

1/2 cup cilantro (chopped)

1 plum tomato

1/2 small onion

1 garlic clove

1 avocado

1/2 lime

1/2 jalapeño

Paprika, to taste

Ground black pepper, to taste

Celtic sea salt, to taste

Raw Taco Meat

1/4 cup walnuts

2 - 3 sundried tomatoes

1/4 teaspoon cumin

1/8 teaspoon garlic powder

1/8 teaspoon smoked paprika

1/8 teaspoon ground white pepper (or ground black pepper)

1/8 teaspoon teaspoon Celtic sea salt

INSTRUCTIONS

1. For *Salad*, rinse, dry and plate lettuce and cilantro. Reserve pinch of cilantro in small mixing bowl.

2. Peel onion and dice. Reserve 1/2 of onion in separate mixing bowl and add remaining onion to reserved cilantro. Remove seeds from jalapeño ad mince. Dice tomato. Add to onion and cilantro with squeeze of lime. Sprinkle on pinch of salt and pepper, and mix to combine. Set aside.

3. Cut avocado in half and remove pit. Scoop flesh into bowl with reserved onion. Peel garlic and mince, and add to avocado with squeeze of lime. Sprinkle on salt, pepper and paprika to taste. Mash slightly and mix with fork until well combine but still chunky. Set aside.

4. For *Raw Taco Meat*, add walnuts, sundried tomatoes, salt, pepper and spices to food processor or high-speed blender. Pulse until coarsely ground.

5. Top *Salad* with *Raw Taco Meat*, avocado and tomato mix. Serve immediately.

Asian Shrimp Lettuce Wraps

Prep Time: 35 minutes

Servings: 2

INGREDIENTS

4 large lettuce leaves (thin, flexible ribs)

1 cup cabbage (shredded)

1 small carrot

1/2 green onion

1/2 inch piece fresh ginger

1 small garlic clove

1/2 teaspoon raw sesame seeds

1/2 teaspoon coconut aminos (or tamari or raw apple cider vinegar)

1 teaspoon raw oil (sesame, coconut, walnut, almond, etc.)

Shrimp

10 - 12 medium shrimp

3/4 cup lemon juice (about 5 lemons)

1 teaspoon red pepper flakes

1/2 green onion (scallion)

Almond Sauce

2 tablespoons raw oil (sesame, coconut, walnut, almond, etc.)

1/4 cup raw almond butter (or 1/2 cup raw almonds)

1 tablespoon lemon juice (or coconut aminos or tamari)

1 tablespoons sweetener*

1/2 small mild chili pepper

Water

INSTRUCTIONS

1. For *Shrimp*, slice green onion and reserve half in small mixing bowl. Peel, devein and remove tails from shrimp. Add to separate bowl with lemon juice, remaining green onion and red pepper. Mix to combine. Shrimp should be completely covered in lemon juice. Place in refrigerator for 30 minutes, or until shrimp are opaque.

2. Peel ginger and garlic, and finely grate or mince. Add to green onion with coconut aminos and oil. Mix to combine. Set aside.

3. For *Almond Sauce*, add oil, almond butter or almonds, lemon juice, sweetener and chili pepper to food processor or high-speed blender. Process until smooth and creamy, about 1 - 2 minutes. Add enough water to reach desired consistency. Transfer to serving dish.

4. Shred cabbage and carrot and add to ginger mixture. Toss to coat.

5. Rinse, dry and plate lettuce leaves. Drain shrimp and layer onto lettuce. Top with cabbage mixture and sprinkle on sesame seeds. Roll up lettuce wraps and serve with *Almond Sauce*.

*stevia, raw honey or dried dates

Savory Stuffed Peppers

Prep Time: 15 minutes

Servings: 1

INGREDIENTS

1 medium-large red bell pepper

1/2 cup cauliflower florets

1/4 small white onion (or sweet onion)

1 celery stalk

1 small carrot

Juice of 1/2 lemon

2 sundried tomatoes

2 tablespoons raw tahini (or 3 tablespoon sesame seeds)

1 tablespoon raw oil (coconut, walnut, almond, sesame, etc.)

1 tablespoon raw pumpkin seeds

1 tablespoon raw sunflower seeds

1 tablespoon dried cranberries (or raisins)

1/2 teaspoon ground cumin

1/4 teaspoon ground ginger

1/4 teaspoon paprika

1/2 teaspoon Celtic sea salt

INSTRUCTIONS

1. Add lemon juice and dried cranberries to medium mixing bowl. Set aside.
2. Slice bell pepper in half and remove seeds and veins. Set aside.

3. Add sundried tomatoes, oil, and tahini or sesame seeds to food processor or high-speed blender. Process until smooth and creamy, about 1 - 2 minutes. Add to cranberries.

4. Add cauliflower and onion to food processor with shredding attachment and process to "rice." Or mince cauliflower and onion. Add to mixing bowl.

5. Finely dice carrot and celery and add to bowl. Add pumpkin seeds, sunflower seeds, salt and spices. Mix to combine.

6. Plate bell pepper halves and stuff with "rice" mixture. Serve immediately.

Veggie Noodle Pad Thai

Prep Time: 10 minutes

Servings: 1

INGREDIENTS

1 medium zucchini

1 large carrot

1 green onion (scallion)

1/2 cup purple cabbage (shredded)

1/2 cup cauliflower florets

1/2 cup mung bean or radish sprouts (optional)

Large bunch cilantro

1/3 cup raw almonds

Raw Pad Thai Sauce

2 tablespoons raw tahini (or 3 tablespoons raw sesame seeds)

2 tablespoons raw nut butter (or 1/4 cup raw nuts)

1 tablespoon lime juice (or lemon juice)

2 tablespoons coconut aminos (or tamari or raw apple cider vinegar)

1 tablespoon sweetener*

1 small garlic clove

1/4 inch piece fresh ginger

INGREDIENTS

1. Use spiralizer, mandolin, vegetable peeler or grater to thinly slice zucchini and carrot. Add to medium bowl. Shred cabbage and slice

green onion. Chop cauliflower and cilantro. Add to bowl with sprouts (optional).

2. Add almonds to food processor or high-speed blender and pulse to coarsely grind. Set aside.

3. For *Raw Pad Thai Sauce*, peel ginger and garlic. Add to food processor or high-speed blender with tahini and nut butter, or sesame seeds and nuts, lime juice, coconut aminos and sweetener. Process until smooth and creamy, about 1 - 2 minutes.

4. Add to veggies and toss to coat. Transfer to serving dish and sprinkle on ground almonds. Serve immediately.

*stevia, raw honey or dried dates

Sweet Coconut Waldorf Salad

Prep Time: 10 minutes

Servings: 2

INGREDIENTS

2 apples

2 celery stalks

2 cups grapes

1 green onion (scallion)

1 small carrot

1 cup raw walnuts (halves or pieces)

1/3 cup raisins (or dried cranberries)

Coconut Cream Dressing

1 coconut

3/4 cup water

2 tablespoons raw walnuts

1 teaspoon mustard seeds

2 tablespoons raw apple cider vinegar (or lemon juice)

1 tablespoons sweetener*

1/2 teaspoon Celtic sea salt

INSTRUCTIONS

1. For *Coconut Cream Dressing*, remove flesh from coconut. Add 1/2 coconut and water to food processor or high-speed blender. Process until well blended and fairly smooth, about 1- 2 minutes.

2. Strain mixture through nut milk bag, cheesecloth or strainer into container. Add coconut milk back to blender with remaining coconut flesh. Process again until well blended and fairly smooth, about 1 minute.

3. Strain mixture again and place coconut cream back into blender. Reserve pulp and set aside to dry and dehydrate, then use as coconut flour.

4. Add walnuts, mustard seeds, vinegar, sweetener and salt to blender and process until smooth, about 1 - 2 minutes. Set aside.

5. Cut grapes in half and add to medium mixing bowl. Dice celery and finely grate carrot. Slice green onion. Add to medium bowl with walnuts and raisins. Seed and stem apples, then dice and add to bowl

6. Add *Coconut Cream Dressing* to bowl and mix to combine. Transfer to serving dishes and serve immediately.

7. Or refrigerate 1 hour and serve chilled

*stevia, raw honey or dried dates

Fresh Sashimi Bento Bowl

Prep Time: 20 minutes*

Servings: 1

INGREDIENTS

2 fresh sea scallops (sushi grade)

2 oz fresh salmon filet (sushi grade)

2 oz fresh tuna filet (sushi grade)

1/2 small cucumber

1/2 avocado

1 sheet nori (dried seaweed/sushi paper)

1/2 lemon

1 oz pickled ginger (or 2 inch piece fresh ginger + 2 tablespoons raw apple cider vinegar and 1 tablespoons raw honey)

1 teaspoon real wasabi (or 2 tablespoons fresh ground horseradish)

1/2 teaspoon raw sesame seeds

2 tablespoons salmon roe or caviar (optional)

Sashimi Sauce

2 teaspoons raw sesame oil (or coconut, walnut, almond oil, etc.)

2 teaspoons coconut aminos (or tamari)

1 - 2 teaspoons raw honey

1/2 small scallion

1/2 piece ginger root

INSTRUCTIONS

1. *For fresh pickled ginger, peel ginger and use mandolin, vegetable peeler or slicing attachment on food processor to thinly slice. Add to glass container with vinegar and honey and refrigerate 1 - 7 days.

2. Have fish monger clean and filet tuna and salmon, and remove skin.

3. Place salmon, tuna and scallops in freezer for about 15 minutes to firm.

4. For sashimi sauce, peel ginger and mince. Slice scallion. Add to small mixing bowl with oil, coconut aminos and honey. Transfer to small serving bowl and set aside.

5. Use spiralizer, mandolin or vegetable peeler to thinly slice cucumber, and arrange around serving dish. Cut avocado in half and slice pitted half in peel. Scoop flesh onto serving dish beside fish.

6. Place pickled ginger and wasabi or horse around serving dish.

7. Slice lemon and cut nori into thin strips. Place around serving dish. Place salmon roe or caviar around serving dish (optional).

8. Remove fish from freezer and thinly slice. Arrange fish in center of serving dish. Serve immediately.

Fresh Clams with Cocktail Sauce

Prep Time: 5 minutes*

Servings: 1

INGREDIENTS

12 large little neck clams

3/4 lemon

Raw Cocktail Sauce

1 large tomato

Juice of 1/4 lemon

2 tablespoons raw sesame seeds(or 1 tablespoon raw tahini)

1 tablespoon fresh ground horseradish

Pinch Celtic sea salt

Pinch cracked black pepper

INSTRUCTIONS

1. Have fishmonger shuck clams. *Or carefully shuck clams yourself.
2. Arrange clams around serving dish.
3. Add sesame seeds to food processor or high-speed blender and process until smooth, if using.
4. Or seed tomato and add to processor or blender with tahini, lemon juice, horseradish, salt and pepper. Process until smooth and transfer to small serving bowl.
5. Serving clams with *Raw Cocktail Sauce* immediately.

Dinner Recipes

Zucchini Pasta with Sundried Tomato Sauce

Prep Time: 5 minutes

Servings: 2

INGREDIENTS

1 large zucchini

Zesty Tomato Sauce

2 medium tomatoes (or 3 plum tomatoes)

5 sundried tomatoes

2 tablespoons raw cashews (or 1 tablespoon raw cashew butter)

2 large garlic cloves

Small bunch fresh basil leaves

1 small fresh oregano sprig

Ground black pepper, to taste

Cayenne pepper, to taste

Celtic sea salt, to taste

INSTRUCTIONS

1. Carefully slice zucchini with spiralizer, vegetable peeler, or sharp knife. Sprinkle with pinch of salt, pepper and cayenne. Gently toss to coat and set aside.

2. For *Zesty Tomato Sauce*, remove basil and oregano leaves from stems. Peel garlic. Add to food processor or high-speed blender

with tomatoes, sundried tomatoes, cashews or cashew butter, salt, pepper and cayenne. Process until smooth, about 1 - 2 minutes.

3. Transfer zucchini pasta to serving dishes. Top with *Zesty Tomato Sauce* and serve immediately.

Zucchini Pasta with Pesto

Prep Time: 10 minutes

Servings: 2

INGREDIENTS

1 small zucchini

1 bell pepper (or 1 carrot)

Pine Nut Pesto

2 1/2 cups fresh basil leaves

1/2 cup raw pine nuts

1 garlic clove

2 tablespoons raw oil (walnut, almond, coconut, sesame, etc.)

1/4 teaspoon ground white pepper (or ground black pepper)

1/4 teaspoon Celtic sea salt

INSTRUCTIONS

1. Carefully slice zucchini with spiralizer, vegetable peeler, or sharp knife. Carefully slice carrot with spiralizer, vegetable peeler, or grater, if using. Or remove stem, seeds and veins from bell pepper, then julienne (cut into long thin slices). Set aside.

2. For *Pine Nut Pesto*, peel garlic and add to food processor or high-speed blender with basil, 2 tablespoons pine nuts, oil, salt and pepper. Process until thick, smooth mixture forms, about 1 - 2 minutes.

3. Add *Pine Nut Pesto* to veggie pasta and toss to coat. Transfer to serving dish and top with remaining pine nuts. Serve immediately.

Zucchini Fettuccini Alfredo

Prep Time: 10 minutes

Servings: 2

INGREDIENTS

1 medium zucchini

1 carrot (or 1 small sweet potato)

Alfredo Sauce

1 cup raw cashews

1 teaspoon lemon juice (or raw apple cider vinegar)

2 garlic cloves

1/2 teaspoon dried thyme

1/2 teaspoon Celtic sea salt

Water

Walnut Parmesan

1/2 cup raw walnuts

3 tablespoons nutritional yeast

1/4 teaspoon ground white pepper (or ground black pepper)

1/2 teaspoon Celtic sea salt

INSTRUCTIONS

1. Carefully slice zucchini and carrot or sweet potato with spiralizer, vegetable peeler, or grater. Set aside.

2. For *Alfredo Sauce*, peel garlic and add to food processor or high-speed blender with cashews, lemon juice, thyme and salt. Process

until smooth mixture forms, up to 5 minutes. Add enough water to reach desired consistency. Set aside.

3. For *Walnut Parmesan*, add walnuts to clean food processor or high-speed blender and process until finely ground. Add nutritional yeast, salt and pepper. Process until coarsely ground and mixture resembling parmesan cheese forms.

4. Add *Alfredo Sauce* to veggie pasta and toss to coat. Transfer to serving dish and top with *Walnut Parmesan*. Serve immediately.

Cashew Crunch Kelp Noodle Salad

Prep Time: 10 minutes*

Servings: 2

INGREDIENTS

1 package (12 oz) kelp noodles

1/2 lemon

1/2 small red bell pepper

Cashew Sauce

1 cup raw cashews

1/2 small red bell pepper

1/2 lemon

1 tablespoon coconut aminos (or raw apple cider vinegar)

2 large basil leaves

1/2 teaspoon smoked paprika

1/2 teaspoon ground black pepper

1/2 teaspoon Celtic sea salt

1/4 teaspoon ground turmeric (optional)

1/4 teaspoon smoked chili powder (optional)

Water

INSTRUCTIONS

1. *Soak 3/4 cup cashews in enough water to cover at least 4 hours, or overnight in refrigerator. Drain and rinse.

2. Drain and rinse kelp noodles. Add to medium bowl with warm water and juice of 1/2 lemon. Set aside 5 minutes.

3. Cut bell pepper in half. Remove stem, seeds and veins and set half of pepper aside. Julienne (thinly slice) remaining bell pepper and add to medium mixing bowl.

5. For *Crunchy Cashew Sauce*, add soaked cashews, bell pepper, juice of 1/2 lemon, coconut aminos, basil, salt and spices to food processor or high-speed blender. Process until smooth, about 2 minutes. Add enough water to reach desired consistency. Set aside.

4. Drain kelp noodles and add to sliced bell pepper. Add *Cashew Sauce* and toss to coat. Transfer noodles to serving dishes.

5. Roughly chop remaining 1/4 cup cashews. Sprinkle noodles and serve immediately. Or refrigerate for 20 minutes and serve chilled.

Tuna Tartar with Avocado and Mango

Prep Time: 15 minutes

Servings: 2

INGREDIENTS

8 oz tuna steak (sushi grade)

1 mango

1 avocado

1 lime

1 garlic clove

Small bunch fresh cilantro

2 tablespoons raw oil (sesame, coconut, almond, walnut, etc.)

1 teaspoon coconut aminos (or raw apple cider vinegar)

1/4 teaspoon red pepper flake

1/4 teaspoon Celtic sea salt

1/4 teaspoon ground pepper

2 tablespoons raw macadamia nuts (optional)

INSTRUCTIONS

1. Add oil, coconut aminos and red pepper flake in small bowl. Cut lime in half and add squeeze of lime. Mix to combine and set aside.

2. Cut avocado in half and remove pit. Dice flesh in peel and scoop into small mixing bowl. Finely chop cilantro. Add to medium mixing bowl with squeeze of remaining lime, salt and pepper. Mix to combine, then set aside.

3. Peel garlic and mince. Cut mango in half around pit. Peel and dice. Add to separate mixing bowl with 1 tablespoon oil and pepper mixture. Toss to coat. Set aside.

4. Dice tuna, discarding any tough white gristle. Finely chop macadamia nuts.

5. Transfer tuna to serving dish. Place in ring mold to form, if preferred. Top with mango and avocado mixtures. Sprinkle on chopped nuts. Drizzle on remaining oil and pepper mixture if preferred.

6. Serve immediately. Or refrigerate 20 minutes and serve chilled.

Raw Walnuts Tacos

Prep Time: 35 minutes

Servings: 2

INGREDIENTS

4 large lettuce leaves (thin, flexible ribs)

1 plum tomato

1/4 red onion (or white or yellow onion)

Medium bunch cilantro

1 avocado

1/2 lime

Taco Meat

1 cup raw walnuts

1/2 cup sundried tomatoes

1/2 teaspoon ground cumin

1/4 teaspoon garlic powder

1/4 teaspoon smoked chili powder

1/4 teaspoon Celtic sea salt

Cayenne pepper, to taste

Cashew Sour Cream

1/2 cup raw cashews

1 lemon

1/8 teaspoon Celtic sea salt

3 tablespoons cup water

1/3 cup ice

INSTRUCTIONS

1. *Soak sundried tomatoes in enough water to cover at least 2 hours, or overnight in refrigerator. Drain.

2. For *Taco Meat*, add soaked tomatoes, walnuts, salt and spices to food processor or high-speed blender. Process until chunky mixture forms, about 1 minute. Set aside

3. For *Cashew Sour Cream*, add cashews, lemon juice, salt, water and ice to clean food processor or high-speed blender. Process until smooth, about 2 minutes.

4. Chop cilantro. Dice tomato. Thinly slice onion. Cut avocado in half, then remove pit and slice in peel.

5. Fill lettuce leaves with *Taco Meat*. Scoop avocado slices onto *Taco Meat*. Drizzle on *Cashew Sour Cream*. Top with diced onion and tomato, and sprinkle of chopped cilantro. Top with squeeze of lime.

6. Fold lettuce around filling and transfer to serving dish. Serve immediately.

Tilapia Lettuce Wraps

Prep Time: 35 minutes

Servings: 2

INGREDIENTS

1 lb boneless, skinless tilapia fillets (or other white fish)

1 1/4 cup lemon juice (about 8 lemons)

4 large lettuce leaves (thin, flexible ribs)

1 cup cabbage (shredded)

1 small carrot

1/2 green onion (scallion)

Cilantro Sauce

1/2 cup raw cashews

1 lemon

1/2 inch piece fresh ginger

1 small garlic clove

Medium bunch cilantro

1/4 teaspoon Celtic sea salt

3 tablespoons water

1/3 cup ice

INSTRUCTIONS

1. Juice lemons into medium mixing bowl. Cut tilapia into 1 inch strips. Add to lemon juice and toss to coat. Tilapia should be completely covered in lemon juice. Place in refrigerator for 30 minutes, or until tilapia is opaque.

2. Carefully slice carrot with spiralizer, vegetable peeler, or grater. Shred cabbage. Slice green onion. Set aside.

3. For *Cilantro Sauce*, remove cilantro leaves form stems. Peel ginger and garlic. Add to food processor or high-speed blender with cashews, lemon juice, salt, water and ice. Process until smooth, about 2 minutes.

4. Remove tilapia from refrigerator and drain. Gently rinse, if preferred. Fill lettuce leaves wit tilapia. Add shredded cabbage and carrot. Drizzle on *Cilantro Sauce*. Top with sliced green onions.

5. Fold lettuce around filling and transfer to serving dish. Serve immediately.

Butternut Squash Soup

Prep Time: 5 minutes

Servings: 2

INGREDIENTS

2 cups butternut squash (chopped)

1/4 cup raw cashews (or 2 tablespoons raw cashew butter or almond butter)

Medium bunch fresh parsley

1/2 avocado

1/4 sweet onion (or white onion)

1 garlic clove

1 inch fresh ginger

1/4 teaspoon ground cinnamon

1/4 teaspoon cayenne pepper

1/4 teaspoon ground cumin

1/4 teaspoon onion powder

1/2 teaspoon curry powder

1/2 teaspoon ground white pepper (or 1/4 teaspoon ground black pepper)

1/2 teaspoon Celtic sea salt

Water

INSTRUCTIONS

1. Cut avocado in half. Scoop flesh of pitted half into food processor or high-speed blender.
2. Peel garlic, ginger and onion. Peel and chop butternut squash. Add to processor with cashews, parsley, salt and spices.

Process until smooth, up to 5 minutes. Add enough water to reach desired consistency.

3. Transfer to serving dish and serve immediately.

Creamy Pumpkin Soup

Prep Time: 5 minutes

Servings: 2

INGREDIENTS

2 cups pumpkin (chopped)

1/4 cup raw cashews (or 2 tablespoon raw cashew butter or almond butter)

1 orange

1 red bell pepper

1/2 avocado

1/4 teaspoon ground cinnamon

1/2 teaspoon ground ginger

1/2 teaspoon Celtic sea salt

1/4 cup raw pumpkin seeds

Water

INSTRUCTIONS

1. Cut avocado in half. Scoop flesh of pitted half into food processor or high-speed blender.

2. Peel and seed orange. Remove stem, seeds and veins from bell pepper. Peel and dice pumpkin. Add to processor with cashews, salt and spices. Process until smooth, up to 5 minutes. Add enough water to reach desired consistency.

3. Transfer to serving dish and top with pumpkin seeds. Serve immediately.

City Clam Chowder

Prep Time: 35 minutes

Servings: 2

INGREDIENTS

2 dozen live littleneck clams

1 - 1 1/2 cups lemon juice (about 8 lemons)

2 cups tomato juice (about 4 large tomatoes)

2 plum tomatoes

1 celery stalk

1 carrot

1 red bell pepper

1 green bell pepper

1/4 teaspoon cayenne pepper

1/2 teaspoon onion powder

1 teaspoon dried oregano

1 teaspoon dried basil

1 teaspoon ground black pepper

1 teaspoon Celtic sea salt

INSTRUCTIONS

1. Have fishmonger shuck clams. Or carefully shuck clams yourself. Reserve clam juice.

2. Juice lemons into medium mixing bowl. Add clams and toss to coat. Clams should be completely covered in lemon juice. Place in refrigerator for 30 minutes, or until clams are opaque.

3. Juice large tomatoes in juicer then add to food processor or high-speed blender. Or add to food processor or high-speed blender and process, then strain and return to processor.

4. Remove stems, seeds and veins from bell peppers. Cut red and green bell pepper in half. Cut carrot and celery stalks in half. Add half of each veggie to tomato juice with salt and spices. Process until smooth, about 2 minutes. Add to medium mixing bowl. Set aside.

5. Dice plum tomatoes, and remaining celery, carrot, and bell pepper. Add to tomato purée with reserved clam juice, salt and spices.

6. Remove clams from refrigerator and drain lemon juice. Gently rinse, if desired. Add to bowl and mix to combine.

7. Transfer to serving dish and serve immediately.

Creamy French Onion Soup

Prep Time: 15 minutes*

Dehydrating Time: 6 hours

Servings: 2

INGREDIENTS

3 cups raw almond milk (or 1 cup raw almonds + 4 cups water)

1/2 lemon

1/4 cup tamari (or coconut aminos or raw apple cider vinegar)

1 tablespoon coconut aminos (or tamari or raw apple cider vinegar)

2 tablespoons raw oil or butter (ghee, cacao butter, coconut butter, almond oil, walnut oil, coconut oil, etc.)

1/2 teaspoon dried thyme

1/2 teaspoon cracked black pepper (or ground black pepper)

Caramelized Onions

2 onions

1 tablespoon raw honey (or 2 dried pitted dates)

1 tablespoon tamari (or coconut aminos or raw apple cider vinegar)

1 tablespoon raw oil (almond, walnut, coconut, etc.)

1/4 teaspoon Celtic sea salt

INSTRUCTIONS

1. *Soak almonds in 1 cup water at least 6 hours, or overnight in refrigerator. Drain and pop off skins, if preferred.

2. For *Caramelized Onions*, add dates, tamari, oil and salt to food processor or high-speed blender and process until smooth. Add water to reach desired consistency, if necessary.

3. Or add honey, tamari, oil and salt to large mixing bowl and mix to combine. Peel onions and thinly slice. Add to bowl and toss to coat.

4. Prepare several dehydrator or parchment sheets and line dehydrator tray. Spread coated onion on prepared trays and place in dehydrator on 110 degrees F for 6 hours.

5. Add soaked almonds to high-speed blender with 3 cups water. Process until well blended and almost smooth, about 1-2 minutes.

6. Strain mixture through nut milk bag, cheesecloth or strainer back into processor. Reserve almond pulp and dehydrate for almond flour.

7. Add juice of 1/2 lemon, coconut aminos, tamari, oil, thyme and black pepper to almond milk. Add half of *Caramelized Onions* and process until smooth, about 1 minute.

8. Add half of remaining *Caramelized Onions* and pulse until onions are roughly chopped.

9. Transfer to serving dish and top with remaining *Caramelized Onions*. Serve immediately.

Salmon Tartar Stack

Prep Time: 10 minutes*

Servings: 2

INGREDIENTS

8 oz boneless, skinless salmon fillet (sushi grade)

2 limes

1 avocado

1 shallot

1 tablespoon raw oil (coconut, walnut, almond, sesame, etc.)

1 teaspoon mustard seeds (or ground mustard)

Medium sprig fresh dill

Celtic sea salt, to taste

Ground black pepper, to taste

2 teaspoons caviar (optional)

INSTRUCTIONS

1. Have fishmonger prepare salmon fillets. Or fillet salmon and remove pin bones and skin.

2. Dice salmon and transfer to serving dish. Top with squeeze of 1/2 lime and sprinkle of salt and pepper. Place in mold to form, if preferred.

3. Peel and thinly slice shallot, then add to small mixing bowl. Juice whole lime into food processor or high-speed blender. Add oil, mustard seeds and pinch of salt and pepper. Process to combine, then add to shallots.

4. Or add lime juice, oil, ground mustard, salt and pepper to shallots. Mix to combine and set aside.

5. Cut avocado in half and remove pit. Dice flesh in peel and scoop into separate mixing bowl. Finely chop dill and add to avocado with squeeze of remaining 1/2 lime, salt and pepper. Mix to combine.

6. Add avocado dill mixture to salmon. Then top with shallot mixture and caviar (optional). Serve immediately.

7. *Or refrigerate 2 hours and serve chilled.

Simple Steak Tartar

Prep Time: 10 minutes*

Servings: 2

INGREDIENTS

10 oz beef tenderloin

Small bunch fresh parsley

1/2 lemon

2 cage-free egg yolk (optional)

2 tablespoons raw oil (coconut, walnut, almond, sesame, etc.)

1 teaspoon ground mustard (or mustard seeds)

1 shallot

1/4 teaspoon chili flakes (optional)

Ground black pepper, to taste

Celtic sea salt, to taste

INSTRUCTIONS

1. Finely dice tenderloin and parsley. Add to bowl with squeeze of lemon and pinch of salt and pepper. Mix to combine.

2. Transfer to serving dish. Place in ring mold to form, if preferred. Set aside.

3. Peel shallot and mince. Add to small mixing bowl with egg yolks (optional), mustard, oil, salt and spices. Whisk to emulsify.

4. Top tenderloin with mixture and serve immediately. Or refrigerate 20 minutes and serve chilled.

Beef Carpaccio with Arugula Salad

Prep Time: 10 minutes*

Servings: 2

INGREDIENTS

10 oz beef tenderloin (top quality)

2 cups fresh baby arugula

1/4 cup raw oil (coconut, walnut, almond, sesame, etc.)

1 cage-free egg yolk

1 teaspoon ground mustard (or mustard seed)

1 lemon

10 cherry or grape tomatoes

Celtic sea salt, to taste

Cracked or ground black pepper, to taste

INSTRUCTIONS

1. *Wrap beef tenderloin in parchment and place in freezer for 1 hour.

2. Remove beef from freezer. Cut against the grain into 1/8 inch thick slices with sharp knife. Place slices between sheets of parchment and gently pound until paper thin with heavy rolling pin or flat end of kitchen mallet.

3. Transfer beef to serving dish and arrange slices to overlap slightly.

4. Rinse, dry and plate arugula. Quarter tomatoes.

5. Add oil, mustard, egg yolk, salt, pepper and squeeze of lemon to food processor or high-speed blender. Process until emulsified, about 1 minute.

6. Top beef slices with baby arugula and drizzle on emulsification. Garnish with tomatoes and serve immediately. Or refrigerate 20 minutes and serve chilled.

Spinach Salad with Shallot Vinaigrette

Prep Time: 5 minutes

Servings: 1

INGREDIENTS

Salad

2 cups spinach leaves

1/4 cup dried cranberries

2 tablespoons raw sunflower seeds

Shallot Vinaigrette

2 shallots

2 tablespoons raw sunflower seeds

2 tablespoons raw apple cider vinegar (or lemon juice)

1/2 teaspoon ground mustard (or mustard seeds)

1 1/2 tablespoons raw oil (coconut, walnut, almond, sesame, etc.)

1/4 teaspoons Celtic sea salt

INSTRUCTIONS

1. For *Salad*, rinse, dry and plate spinach. Sprinkle dried cranberries and sunflowers seeds over greens.

2. For *Shallot Vinaigrette*, peel and chop shallots. Add to food processor or high-speed blender with vinegar, sunflower seeds, mustard, oil and salt. Process until smooth, about 1 minute.

3. Drizzle *Shallot Vinaigrette* over salad and serve immediately.

Awesome Oysters

Prep Time: 5 minutes*

Servings: 1

INGREDIENTS

12 large fresh oysters

1 lemon

3 tablespoons caviar

1 inch piece fresh horseradish root (or 1 teaspoon fresh ground horseradish)

Pinch Celtic sea salt

Pinch cracked black pepper

INSTRUCTIONS

1. Have fishmonger shuck oysters. *Or carefully shuck oysters yourself.
2. Arrange oysters on serving dish.
3. Cut lemon in half and squeeze juice over oysters. Use microplane or small grater to finely grate fresh radish over oysters. Sprinkle salt and pepper to taste over oysters.
4. Top oysters with small dollop of fresh caviar and serve immediately.

Dill Stuffed Tomatoes

Prep Time: 15 minutes*

Servings: 2

INGREDIENTS

4 medium tomatoes

1 celery stalk

1 small carrot

1 green onion (scallion)

1/3 cup sunflower seeds

1/2 red bell pepper

1/4 small red onion (or sweet onion)

1/2 teaspoon Celtic sea salt

Dill Dressing

1/2 cup raw cashews

1 tablespoon raw apple cider vinegar (or coconut aminos)

1 teaspoon ground mustard (or mustard seeds)

1/2 lemon

1 small garlic clove

2 sprigs fresh dill

1/2 teaspoon Celtic sea salt

1/4 teaspoon ground white pepper (or pinch ground black pepper)

Water

INSTRUCTIONS

1. *Soak cashews in enough water to cover at least 4 hours, or overnight in refrigerator. Drain and rinse.

2. Cut tops off tomatoes and scoop out seeds. Set aside.

3. Finely dice celery and carrot. Slice green onion. Peel and dice onion. Add to medium mixing bowl. Remove stem, seeds and veins from bell pepper, then dice. Add to bowl with sprinkle of salt. Set aside.

4. For *Dill Dressing*, peel garlic and add to food processor or high-speed blender with soaked cashews, vinegar, mustard, squeeze of lemon, dill, salt and pepper. Process until smooth and creamy, about 1 - 2 minutes. Add enough water to reach desired consistency.

5. Pour *Dill Dressing* over chopped veggies. Toss to coat.

6. Plate hollowed tomatoes and stuff with *Dill Dressing* veggie mixture. Serve immediately.

Savory Stuffed Portobello

Prep Time: 35 minutes

Dehydrating Time: 1 hour

Servings: 2

INGREDIENTS

2 large Portobello mushrooms

2 tablespoons raw oil (walnut, almond, coconut, sesame, etc.)

1 tablespoon coconut aminos (or raw apple cider vinegar or tamari)

1 cup macadamia nuts

1 cup spinach

Medium bunch fresh parsley

1/3 cup sundried tomatoes

1 small lemon

1 garlic clove

1 tablespoon nutritional yeast

1 tablespoon water

1/2 teaspoon ground white pepper (or 1/4 teaspoon ground black pepper)

1/4 teaspoon Celtic sea salt

INSTRUCTIONS

1. *Soak macadamia nuts in enough water to cover at least 2 hours, or overnight in refrigerator. Soak sundried tomatoes in enough water to cover at least 4 hours, or overnight in refrigerator, if tough and chewy. Drain.

2. Cut stems off of mushrooms, if present. Chop stems and add to small mixing bowl.

3. Scrape gills from inside mushroom cap with spoon. Clean mushroom caps with damp towel. Pat dry. Add to mixing bowl with oil and coconut aminos. Toss to coat and set aside 30 - 40 minutes. Toss to coat frequently while marinating.

4. Peel garlic. Juice lemon. Add to food processor or high-speed blender with soaked tomatoes, nutritional yeast, water, salt and pepper. Process until fairly smooth, about 2 minutes.

5. Add parsley and spinach. Pulse to roughly chop greens. Mix in marinated mushroom stems, if present.

6. Line dehydrator tray with dehydrator or parchment sheet.

7. Fill mushroom caps with mixture and place on prepared dehydrator tray. Dehydrate on 105 degrees F for 1 hour.

8. Transfer to serving dish and serve immediately.

Garlic Almond Bread

Prep Time: 35 minutes

Dehydrating Time: 16 hours

Servings: 12

INGREDIENTS

2 cups ground almonds

1 cup psyllium husk powder

1 cup young coconut flesh

1/2 cup ground flax seed

3 dried pitted dates

4 garlic cloves

2 teaspoons garlic powder

1/2 lemon

1/2 teaspoon dried parsley

1/2 teaspoon ground black pepper

1 teaspoon Celtic sea salt

INSTRUCTIONS

1. Pry coconut flesh away from peel. Peel garlic. Add to food
   processor or high-speed blender with dates, lemon juice, garlic
   powder, parsley, salt and pepper. Process until finely ground, about
   2 minutes.

2. Add ground almonds, psyllium husk and ground flax. Process until
   well combined, about 1 minute.

3. Line dehydrator tray with dehydrator or parchment sheet.

4. Form mixture into 2 loaves and place on lined dehydrator tray. Dehydrate on 115 degrees F for 12 - 16 hours.

5. Remove from dehydrator and slice. Transfer to serving dish and serve immediately. Or store in refrigerator up to 4 days.

Gyro Wrap with Avocado Tzatziki

Prep Time: 20 minutes*

Dehydrating Time: 15 hours

Servings: 4

INGREDIENTS

2 romaine lettuce leaves

1 large tomato

1/4 small white onion

Pita Bread

1 cup golden flax seeds

1/2 avocado

1/2 teaspoon Celtic sea salt

Water

Gyro Meat

1 1/2 cups raw walnuts

1/4 small white onion

2 garlic cloves

1 teaspoon ground cumin

1 teaspoon ground dried rosemary (or 1/2 sprig fresh rosemary)

1 teaspoon ground dried thyme

1/2 teaspoon dried oregano

1/2 teaspoon ground black pepper

1/2 teaspoon dried marjoram (optional)

1/2 teaspoon Celtic sea salt

Water

Avocado Tzatziki

1/2 small cucumber

1/2 avocado

1 teaspoon lemon juice

1/2 teaspoon apple cider vinegar (optional)

1 garlic clove

2 mint leaves

1/8 teaspoon Celtic sea salt

INSTRUCTIONS

1. *For *Pita Bread*, soak flax in 1 cup water for 6 hours.
2. Cut avocado in half. Scoop flesh of pitted half into food processor or high-speed blender. Add soaked flax and salt. Process until finely ground and well combined, about 2 minutes. Preserve remaining avocado half with pit in air tight container.
3. Prepare dehydrator trays with dehydrator or parchment sheets. Evenly spread 1/3 cup portions of batter on sheets in 1/8 inch thick circles.
4. Dehydrate at 105 degrees F for 3 hours. Flip bread over, remove sheet and continue dehydrating for 2 hours. Remove bread from the dehydrator and allow to rest for several hours to become more flexible, in zip top plastic bag if preferred.
5. *For *Gyro Meat*, soak walnuts in enough water to cover at least 4 hours, or overnight in refrigerator. Drain.

6. Peel onion and add to clean food processor or high-speed blender with soaked walnuts, salt and spices. Process until chunky mixture forms, about 1 minute.

7. Line dehydrator tray with dehydrator or parchment sheet.

8. Form mixture into loaf and flatten to 1/4 inch thick sheet. Place on lined dehydrator tray. Dehydrate on 110 degrees F for 8 - 10 hours.

9. Remove from dehydrator and slice into 1 x 6 inch strips. Set aside.

10. For *Avocado Tzatziki*, peel and mince garlic. Mince mint. Peel, seed and shred or grate cucumber. Add to small mixing bowl. Remove pit from avocado half and scoop flesh into small mixing bowl. Add lemon juice, salt and vinegar (optional). Mix well.

11. Cut tomato in half and remove seeds. Chop tomato, lettuce and onion.

12. Transfer *Pita Bread* to serving dish. Fill with *Gyro Meat* strips. Top with *Avocado Tzatziki*, and chopped tomato, lettuce and onion. Fold *Pita Bread* over filling and serve immediately.

Savory Nut Meatloaf

Prep Time: 5 minutes*

Dehydrating Time: 4 hours

Servings: 2

INGREDIENTS

Meatloaf

1 cup raw walnuts

1 cup raw sunflower seeds

1 cup raw almonds

1 small celery stalk

1 large red bell pepper

1 small chili pepper (jalapeño, Serrano, etc.)

1/4 small onion

2 garlic cloves

Large bunch fresh parsley

2 springs fresh rosemary

1 tablespoon fresh cumin (or 1 teaspoon ground cumin)

1 teaspoon Celtic sea salt

Water

Raw Ketchup

1 plum tomato

1/4 cup sundried tomatoes

2 - 3 dried pitted dates (or 2 tablespoons raw honey)

2 teaspoons raw apple cider vinegar

1/4 teaspoon Celtic sea salt

Pinch onion powder

Pinch garlic powder

INSTRUCTIONS

1. *For *Meatloaf*, soak walnuts, almonds and sunflower seeds in enough water to cover for 2 hours. Drain.

2. For *Raw Ketchup*, soak sundried tomatoes and dates (if using) in enough water to cover for at least 1 hour. Drain and reserve 2 teaspoons soaking liquid.

3. Add soaked sundried tomatoes and dates, reserved liquid, plum tomato, vinegar, salt, spices and honey (if using) to food processor or high-speed blender. Process until smooth, about 1 - 2 minutes. Set aside.

4. Peel garlic. Remove seeds, stems and veins from bell and chili peppers. Peel onion. Chop garlic, peppers, celery, onion, parsley and rosemary. Add to food processor or high-speed blender with soaked nuts, cumin and salt. Process until well ground, about 2 minutes. Add enough water to reach desired consistency.

5. Line dehydrator tray with dehydrator or parchment sheet.

6. Form mixture into loaf and place on lined dehydrator tray. Dehydrate on 110 degrees F for 1 hour. Remove loaf and top with *Raw Ketchup*. Continue dehydrating for 3 hours.

7. Remove from dehydrator and slice. Transfer to serving dish and top with more *Raw Ketchup*, if preferred. Serve immediately.

Tuscan Rustic Pizza

Prep Time: 25 minutes*

Servings: 2

INGREDIENTS

Pizza Crust

1 cup flax seeds (or 1/2 cup flax seeds + 1/2 cup chia seeds)

1 cup raw sunflower seeds

2 tablespoons raw oil (coconut, walnut, almond, sesame, etc.)

2 teaspoons dries oregano

1/4 teaspoon Celtic sea salt

Water

Pizza Sauce

1 plum tomato

2 large basil leaves

1/2 teaspoon dried oregano (or 1 teaspoon fresh oregano)

1/8 teaspoon Celtic sea salt

Macadamia Cheese

1 cup raw macadamia nuts

1/2 shallot

1 teaspoon lemon juice

1/4 teaspoon Celtic sea salt

Water

Toppings

1/2 red bell pepper

1/2 yellow bell pepper

1/4 cup grape tomatoes

1/4 white or sweet onion

Small bunch fresh basil

INSTRUCTIONS

1. *For *Macadamia Cheese*, soak nuts in enough water to cover overnight in refrigerator. Drain and rinse.

2. Peel shallot. Add to food processor or high-speed blender with soaked macadamia nuts, lemon juice, and salt. Process until smooth, up to 5 minutes. Add enough water to reach desired consistency. Set aside.

3. For *Pizza Crust*, add flax and sunflower seeds to food processor or high-speed blender. Process until finely ground. Add oregano and oil. Pulse to combine,

4. Place mixture in large mixing bowl or on parchment lined cutting board and knead in enough water to reach desired consistency. Press dough into bottom of serving dish. Set aside.

5. For *Pizza Sauce*, add tomato, basil, oregano and salt to clean food processor or high-speed blender. Process until smooth, about 1 minute. Set aside.

6. For *Toppings*, cut bell peppers in half and remove seed, stems and veins. Peel onion, Thinly slice bell pepper, onion and fresh basil. Cut grape tomatoes in half.

7. Spread *Pizza Sauce* over *Pizza Crust*. Top *Pizza Sauce* with *Macadamia Cheese*. Sprinkle with *Toppings*. Slice and serve immediately.

Zucchini Mac and Cashew Cheese

Prep Time: 10 minutes

Servings: 2

INGREDIENTS

1 large zucchini

1/2 teaspoon ground black pepper

Cheese Sauce

1 cup raw cashews

1/2 red bell pepper

1/3 cup nutritional yeast

1 tablespoon coconut aminos (or raw apple cider vinegar)

1/2 lemon

1/2 teaspoon smoked chili powder

1/4 teaspoonCeltic sea salt

Water

Almond Parmesan

1/2 cup raw almonds (or walnuts, cashews, etc.)

3 tablespoons nutritional yeast

1/2 teaspoon Celtic sea salt

1/2 teaspoon ground white pepper (or ground black pepper)

INSTRUCTIONS

1. *Soak cashews in enough water to cover at least 4 hours, or overnight in refrigerator. Drain and rinse.

2. Carefully slice zucchini with spiralizer, vegetable peeler, or shredding attachment on food processor. Add to medium mixing bowl with black pepper. Toss to coat and set aside.

3. Four *Cheese Sauce*, cut bell pepper in half and remove seeds, stems and veins. Add to food processor or high-speed blender with soaked cashews, nutritional yeast, coconut aminos, lemon juice, chili powder and salt. Process until smooth, about 1 - 2 minutes. Add enough water to reach desired consistency, if necessary.

4. For *Almond Parmesan*, add almonds to clean food processor or high-speed blender and process until finely ground. Add nutritional yeast, salt and pepper. Process until coarsely ground and mixture resembling parmesan cheese forms.

5. Add *Cheese Sauce* to zucchini and toss to coat. Transfer to serving dish and top with *Almond Parmesan* and crack black pepper, if preferred. Serve immediately.

Squash Blossom Stuffers

Prep Time: 10 minutes*

Servings: 4

INGREDIENTS

16 squash blossoms

1/2 cup walnuts

1 avocado

1 small onion

1/2 sprig fresh dill

1/2 lemon

1/2 teaspoon dried thyme

1/2 teaspoon ground white pepper (or ground black pepper)

1/2 teaspoon Celtic sea salt

1 teaspoon dried tarragon (optional)

Water

INSTRUCTIONS

1. *Gently rinse blossoms and pat dry. Let air dry for 30 minutes.

2. Cut avocado in half and remove pit. Scoop flesh into food processor or high-speed blender with walnuts, dill, squeeze of lemon, salt, pepper and spices. Process until smooth, about 2 minutes. Add enough water to reach desired consistency.

3. Peel onion and mince. Add to small mixing bowl with avocado mixture. Mix to combine.

4. Spoon mixture into squash blossoms. Serve immediately.

Zucchini Walnut Lasagna

Prep Time: 15 minutes*

Servings: 4

INGREDIENTS

1 medium zucchini

Sundried Marinara

1 cup sundried tomatoes

1 plum tomato

1 dried pitted date

2 tablespoons raw oil (coconut, walnut, almond, sesame, etc.)

1 garlic clove

1/2 lemon

1/2 teaspoon dried basil

1/2 teaspoon dried oregano

1/4 teaspoon ground black pepper

Spinach Pesto

3 cups spinach

1/2 cup raw walnuts

1/4 cup raw oil (coconut, walnut, almond, sesame, etc.)

2 garlic cloves

1/2 lemon

Cashew Cheese

3/4 cup raw cashews

1 garlic clove

1 teaspoon lemon juice

1/4 Celtic sea salt

Walnut Sausage

2 cups raw walnuts

2 tablespoons coconut aminos (or tamari or raw apple cider vinegar)

1 teaspoon dried sage

1 teaspoon dried thyme

1 teaspoon fresh rosemary

1 teaspoon dried marjoram (optional)

1/2 teaspoon Celtics sea salt

INSTRUCTIONS

1. * Separately soak cashews, walnuts, and sundried tomatoes and date in enough water to cover at least 6 hours, or overnight in refrigerator. Drain and rinse nuts. Drain sundried tomatoes and date.

2. For *Sundried Marinara*, peel garlic and add to food processor or high-speed blender with soaked tomatoes and date, fresh tomato, oil, spices and squeeze of lemon. Process until finely ground and fairly smooth, about 1 - 2 minutes. Add enough water to reach desired consistency, if necessary. Set aside.

3. For *Spinach Pesto*, peel garlic and add to clean food processor or high-speed blender with soaked walnuts, spinach, oil and squeeze of lemon. Process until finely ground, about 2 minutes. Add enough water or oil to reach desired consistency, if necessary. Set aside.

4. Four *Cashew Cheese*, peel garlic and add to clean food processor or high-speed blender with soaked cashews, salt and lemon juice. Process until smooth, about 2 minutes. Add enough water to reach desired consistency, if necessary. Set aside.

5. For *Walnut Sausage*, add soaked walnuts, coconut aminos, salt and spices to clean food processor or high-speed blender. Process until coarsely ground, about 1 minute. Set aside.

6. Carefully slice zucchini into 1/8 - 1/4 inch long strips with knife or mandolin. Place layer of zucchini on serving dish. Alternate layers of *Sundried Marinara* and *Cashew Cheese*, and layers of *Spinach Pesto* and *Walnut Sausage* with zucchini layers. End with *Walnut Sausage*.

7. Slice and serve immediately. Or place inn refrigerator for 20 minute and serve chilled.

Dessert Recipes

Sweet Banana Cream pie

Prep Time: 10 minutes*

Servings: 8

INGREDIENTS

Crust

1 cup raw cashews

1 cup flaked or shredded coconut

1/2 cup dried pitted dates

1/4 teaspoon vanilla

1/4 teaspoon Celtic sea salt

Banana Filling

2 ripe bananas

3/4 cup raw cashews (or 1/2 cup raw cashew butter)

1/3 cup raw coconut oil (or raw coconut or cacao butter, melted)

1/4 cup raw honey (or dried pitted dates, soaked overnight)

Juice of 2 lemons

1 teaspoon vanilla

Pinch Celtic sea salt

Water (optional)

INSTRUCTIONS

1. *For *Banana Filling*, soak dates in enough water to cover overnight in refrigerator, if using. Drain.

2. For *Crust,* place all ingredients in food processor or high-speed blender. Process until well ground and mixture sticks together, about 1 - 2 minutes.

3. Press *Crust* firmly into pie plate, cake pan or baking dish with hands.

4. For *Banana Filling,* peel bananas and juice lemons. Add to clean food processor or high-speed blender with cashews or cashew butter, coconut oil or butter, vanilla, salt and honey or soaked dates. Process until creamy and smooth, about 1 - 2 minutes.

5. Pour *Banana Filling* into *Crust* and smooth with spatula or back of a spoon.

6. *Cover pie with parchment, if preferred, and place in freezer at least 8 hours, or overnight.

7. Slice and serve chilled. Or allow to soften slightly, then serve. Store leftovers in freezer.

Creamy Chocolate Pie

Prep Time: 15 minutes*

Servings: 8

INGREDIENTS

Crust

1 cup dried pitted dates

3/4 cup raw almonds

1/2 cup raw walnuts

3 tablespoons raw cocoa powder

1/2 teaspoon vanilla

1/4 teaspoon Celtic sea salt

Water

Chocolate Cream Filling

4 cups raw cashews

1/2 cup raw honey (or 1 cup dried pitted dates)

1/4 cup raw cocoa powder

3 teaspoons vanilla

2 tablespoons cacao nibs (or raw chocolate chips or raw chocolate bark)

Water

INSTRUCTIONS

1. *For *Crust*, soak dates in enough water to cover for 1 hour, then drain.

2. *For *Chocolate Cream Filling*, soak cashews in enough water to cover overnight in refrigerator. Drain and rinse. Set aside. Soak

dates in enough water to cover overnight in refrigerator, if using. Drain, reserving soaking liquid.

3. For *Crust*, place all ingredients in food processor or high-speed blender. Process until well ground and mixture sticks together, about 2 minutes.

4. Press *Crust* firmly into pie plate, cake pan or baking dish with hands. Set aside in refrigerator or freezer, if preferred.

5. For *Chocolate Cream Filling*, add soaked cashews, vanilla, and dates or honey to clean food processor or high-speed blender. Process until smooth, about 2 minutes. Add enough date soaking liquid or water to reach desired consistency. Mixture should be thick and smooth, but not runny.

6. Transfer half of mixture to small mixing bowl and set aside. Add cocoa to processor and process until incorporated.

7. Pour *Chocolate Cream Filling* into *Crust* and smooth with spatula or back of a spoon. Top with reserved *Cream Filling* and smooth with spatula or back of a spoon. Chop cacao nibs, or shave chocolate bark. Sprinkle chopped nibs, chocolate shaving or chocolate chips over pie.

8. *Refrigerate or freeze at least 1 hour, until set. Slice and serve chilled.

Lemon Chiffon Pie

Prep Time: 15 minutes*

Servings: 8

INGREDIENTS

Crust

2 cups raw almonds

1/2 cup dried pitted dates

1/4 cup flaked or shredded coconut

Lemon Cheesecake Filling

3 cups raw cashews

3/4 cup fresh lemon juice (about 6 lemons)

3/4 cup raw honey (or 1 cup dried pitted dates)

3/4 cup raw coconut oil (or raw coconut or cacao butter, melted)

1 teaspoon vanilla

1/2 teaspoon Celtic sea salt

INSTRUCTIONS

1. *For *Crust*, soak almonds in enough water to cover overnight in refrigerator. Drain and rinse.

2. *For *Lemon Cheesecake Filling*, soak cashews in enough water to cover for 4 hours. Drain and rinse. Set aside. Soak dates in enough water to cover overnight in refrigerator, if using. Drain, reserving soaking liquid.

3. For *Crust*, place all ingredients in food processor or high-speed blender. Process until well ground and mixture sticks together, about 2 minutes.

4. Press *Crust* firmly into pie plate, cake pan or baking dish with hands. Set aside in refrigerator or freezer, if preferred.

5. For *Lemon Cheesecake Filling*, zest 1 lemon, then juice all lemons into clean food processor or high-speed blender. Add soaked cashews, vanilla, coconut oil or butter, salt, and honey or dates to clean food processor or high-speed blender. Process until smooth, about 2 - 3 minutes. Add enough date soaking liquid or water to reach desired consistency, if necessary. Mixture should be thick and smooth, but not runny.

6. Pour *Lemon Cheesecake Filling* into *Crust* and gently tap dish on counter to release any air bubbles. Smooth with spatula or back of a spoon, if needed.

7. *Cover pie with parchment, if preferred, and place in freezer at least 3 hours. Allow to warm slightly and serve chilled.

Key Lime Cream Pie

Prep Time: 15 minutes*

Servings: 8

INGREDIENTS

Crust

1 cup raw macadamia nuts

1 cup raw cashews

1/3 cup flaked or shredded coconut

1/4 cup dried pitted dates

1 teaspoon vanilla

1/2 teaspoon Celtic sea salt

Key Lime Filling

1 1/2 cups raw cashews

1 ripe avocado

3/4 cup key lime juice (about 8 key limes)

3/4 cup raw honey (or 1 cup dried pitted dates)

1/4 cup raw coconut oil (or raw coconut or cacao butter, melted)

1 tablespoon vanilla

1/4 teaspoon Celtic sea salt

1/2 teaspoon spirulina or spinach powder (optional)

INSTRUCTIONS

1. *For *Key Lime Filling*, soak cashews in enough water to cover for 1 hour. Drain and rinse. Set aside. Soak dates in enough water to

cover overnight in refrigerator, if using. Drain, reserving soaking liquid.

2. For *Crust*, place all ingredients in food processor or high-speed blender. Process until well ground and mixture sticks together, about 2 minutes.

3. Press *Crust* firmly into pie plate, cake pan or baking dish with hands. Set aside in refrigerator or freezer, if preferred.

4. For *Key Lime Filling*, zest 1 lime, then juice all limes into clean food processor or high-speed blender. Cut avocado in half and scoop flesh into processor.

5. Add soaked cashews, coconut oil or butter, honey or soaked dates, vanilla, salt and spirulina and spinach powder (optional). Process until smooth, about 2 - 3 minutes. Add enough date soaking liquid or water to reach desired consistency, if necessary. Mixture should be thick and smooth, but not runny.

6. Pour *Key Lime Filling* into *Crust* and gently tap dish on counter to release any air bubbles. Smooth with spatula or back of a spoon, if needed.

7. *Cover pie with parchment, if preferred, and place in freezer at least 3 hours. Allow to warm slightly and serve chilled.

Coconut Cream Pie

Prep Time: 20 minutes*

Servings: 8

INGREDIENTS

Crust

3/4 cup raw macadamia nuts

3/4 cup raw almonds

1/2 cup dried pitted dates

1/2 cup flaked or shredded coconut

Coconut Cream Filling

1 1/2 cups raw cashews

1 1/2 cups flaked or shredded coconut

3/4 cup raw honey (or 1 cup dried pitted dates))

3/4 cup raw coconut oil (or coconut or cacao butter, melted)

1 teaspoon vanilla

1/2 teaspoon Celtic sea salt

Water

INSTRUCTIONS

1. *For *Crust*, soak almonds in enough water to cover overnight in refrigerator. Drain and rinse.

2. *For *Coconut Cream Filling*, soak cashews in enough water to cover for 4 hours. Drain and rinse. Set aside. Soak coconut in 2 cups water overnight in refrigerator. Drain, reserving soaking

liquid. Soak dates in enough water to cover overnight in refrigerator, if using. Drain, reserving soaking liquid.

3. For *Crust*, place all ingredients in food processor or high-speed blender. Process until well ground and mixture sticks together, about 2 minutes.

4. Press *Crust* firmly into pie plate, cake pan or baking dish with hands. Set aside in refrigerator or freezer, if preferred.

6. For *Coconut Cream Filling*, add soaked coconut to clean food processor or high-speed blender. Process until smooth and creamy, up to 5 minutes. Scrape down sides of bowl as necessary.

5. Add soaked cashews, vanilla, coconut oil or butter, salt, and honey or dates to processor. Process until smooth, about 2 - 3 minutes. Add enough date and/or coconut soaking liquid or water to reach desired constancy, if necessary. Mixture should be thick and smooth, but not runny.

6. Pour *Coconut Cream Filling* into *Crust* and gently tap dish on the counter to release any air bubbles. Smooth with spatula or back of a spoon, if needed.

7. *Cover pie with parchment, if preferred, and place in freezer at least 3 hours. Allow to warm slightly and serve chilled.

Simple Pecan Pie

Prep Time: 15 minutes*

Servings: 8

INGREDIENTS

Crust

3/4 cup raw pecans

3/4 cup raw walnuts

1 1/4 cups dried pitted dates

1/4 cup flaked or shredded coconut

1/4 teaspoon Celtic sea salt

Pecan Filling

1 2/3 cups dried pitted dates

1/2 raw pecan pieces (or 3/4 raw pecan halves)

3/4 cup raw pecan halves (reserve)

1/4 cup raw coconut oil (or raw coconut or cacao butter, melted)

1 1/2 teaspoons vanilla

1 teaspoon ground cinnamon

1/4 teaspoon ground nutmeg

1/2 teaspoon Celtic sea salt

Water

INSTRUCTIONS

1. *For *Pecan Filling,* soak dates in enough water to cover for at least 4 hours, or overnight in refrigerator. Drain, reserving soaking liquid .

2. For *Crust*, place all ingredients in food processor or high-speed blender. Process until mixture is well ground and sticks together, about 2 - 3 minutes.

3. Press *Crust* firmly into pie plate, cake pan or baking dish with hands. Set aside in refrigerator or freezer, if preferred.

4. For *Pecan Filling*, add soaked dates to clean food processor or high-speed blender with pecan pieces, coconut oil or butter, vanilla, salt and spices. Process until thick smooth mixture forms, about 2 - 3 minutes. Add enough soaking liquid to reach desired consistency.

5. Pour *Pecan Filling* into *Crust* and smooth with spatula or back of a spoon. Top pie with reserve pecan halves.

6. Slice and serve immediately. Or refrigerate at least 1 hour and serve chilled.

Modern Mincemeat Pie

Prep Time: 15 minutes*

Servings: 8

INGREDIENTS

Crust

1 cup raw almonds

1 cup raw pecans

1 cup raw walnuts

1 1/2 cups dried pitted dates

1/2 orange

1/2 teaspoon vanilla

1/2 teaspoon ground cinnamon

1/4 teaspoon ground nutmeg

1/4 teaspoon Celtic sea salt

Mincemeat Filling

2 cups dried pitted dates

1/2 cup raw almonds

1/2 cup dried apricots

1 1/2 oranges

1/2 lemon

2 tablespoons raw tahini

2 tablespoons raisins

2 tablespoons dried cherries (or goji or noni berries)

2 tablespoons raw pistachios

2 tablespoons shredded or flaked coconut

1 tablespoon chia seeds

1 teaspoon vanilla

1 teaspoon ground cinnamon

1/4 teaspoon ground nutmeg

1/4 teaspoon ground ginger

1/4 teaspoon Celtic sea salt

Water

INSTRUCTIONS

1. *For *Mincemeat Filling,* soak dates in enough water to cover for 1 hour, then drain.

2. For *Crust*, zest then juice orange into food processor or high-speed blender. Add all *Crust* ingredients and process until well ground and mixture sticks together, about 2 - 3 minutes.

3. Press *Crust* firmly into pie plate, cake pan or baking dish with hands. Set aside in refrigerator or freezer, if preferred.

4. For *Mincemeat Filling*, add chia to clean food processor or high-speed blender and process until finely ground, about 1 minute. Add raw almonds and process until finely ground, about 2 minutes.

5. Zest *then* juice oranges and lemon. Add to processor with soaked dates, tahini, salt and spices. Process until well ground and fairly smooth, about 2 minutes. Add apricots and pulse until roughly chopped.

6. Transfer to medium mixing bowl and stir in raisins and cherries. Mix to combine.

7. Pour *Mincemeat Filling* into *Crust* and smooth with spatula or back of a spoon. Roughly chop pistachios. Sprinkle chopped pistachios and coconut over pie.

8. Slice and serve immediately. Or refrigerate at least 1 hour and serve chilled.

Holiday Pumpkin Pie

Prep Time: 15 minutes*

Servings: 8

INGREDIENTS

Crust

3/4 cup raw pecans

3/4 cup raw walnuts

1 1/4 cups dried pitted dates

Pinch Celtic sea salt

Pumpkin Filling

1 "pie pumpkin"

1 1/2 cups dried pitted dates

1/2 cup dried apricots

2 teaspoons ground cinnamon

1/2 teaspoon ground ginger

1/2 teaspoon vanilla

Water

INSTRUCTIONS

1. *For *Crust*, soak dates in enough water to cover for 1 hour, then drain.
2. *For *Pumpkin Filling,* soak dates in enough water to cover for at least 4 hours, or overnight in refrigerator. Drain, reserving soaking liquid .

3. For *Crust*, place all ingredients in food processor or high-speed blender. Process until mixture is well ground and sticks together, about 2 - 3 minutes.

4. Press *Crust* firmly into pie plate, cake pan or baking dish with hands. Set aside in refrigerator or freezer, if preferred.

5. For *Pumpkin Filling*, peel pumpkin and remove seeds and stringy innards. Chop pumpkin and add to clean food processor or high-speed blender with soaked dates, apricots, vanilla, cinnamon and ginger. Process until smooth, up to 5 minutes. Add enough soaking liquid to reach desired consistency. Mixture should be thick and smooth, but not runny.

6. Pour *Pumpkin Filling* into *Crust* and smooth with spatula or back of a spoon.

7. Slice and serve immediately. Or refrigerate at least 1 hour and serve chilled.

Creamy Strawberry Cheesecake

Prep Time: 15 minutes*

Servings: 8

INGREDIENTS

Crust

1 cup raw macadamia nuts

1/2 cup raw walnuts

1/2 cup dried pitted dates

1/4 cup flaked or shredded coconut

Strawberry Cheesecake Filling

2 1/2 cups raw cashews

2 cups strawberries (fresh or thawed)

1/2 cup raw honey (or dried pitted dates)

1/2 cup raw coconut oil (or raw coconut or cacao butter, melted)

1 teaspoon vanilla

INSTRUCTIONS

1. *For *Strawberry Cheesecake Filling*, soak cashews in enough water to cover for 4 hours. Drain and rinse. Set aside. Soak dates in enough water to cover overnight in refrigerator, if using. Drain, reserving soaking liquid.

2. For *Crust*, place all ingredients in food processor or high-speed blender. Process until well ground and mixture sticks together, about 2 minutes.

3. Press *Crust* firmly into pie plate, cake pan or baking dish with hands. Set aside in refrigerator or freezer, if preferred.

4. For *Strawberry Cheesecake Filling*, remove stems from fresh strawberries, or thaw frozen strawberries. Add to clean food processor or high-speed blender with soaked cashews, honey or soaked dates, coconut oil or butter, and vanilla. Process until smooth, about 2 - 3 minutes. Add enough date soaking liquid or water to reach desired consistency, if necessary. Mixture should be thick and smooth, but not runny.

5. Pour *Strawberry Cheesecake Filling* into *Crust* and gently tap dish on counter to release any air bubbles. Smooth with spatula or back of a spoon, if needed.

6. *Cover pie with parchment, if preferred, and place in freezer at least 2 hours. Allow to warm slightly and serve chilled.

Lemon Curd Dessert Tart

Prep Time: 10 minutes*

Servings: 8

INGREDIENTS

1 1/2 cups fresh blueberries

Tart Shell

1 cup raw cashews (or raw walnuts)

1 cup raw macadamia nuts (or raw brazil nuts)

1/3 cup flaked or shredded coconut

1 cup dried pitted dates

1/2 teaspoon vanilla

Lemon Curd Filling

1 cup cashews

1/2 cup raw coconut butter (or raw cacao butter)

4 lemons

1/3 - 1/2 cup raw honey (or dried pitted dates)

Pinch Celtic sea salt

Pinch vanilla (optional)

Pinch ground turmeric (optional)

Water

INSTRUCTIONS

1. *For *Lemon Curd Filling*, soak cashews in enough water to cover at least 4 hours, or overnight in refrigerator. Drain and

rinse. Set aside. Soak dates in enough water to cover overnight in refrigerator, if using. Drain, reserving soaking liquid.

2. For *Tart Shell*, place all ingredients in food processor or high-speed blender. Process until well ground and mixture sticks together, about 2 minutes.

3. Press *Crust* firmly into tart pan or pie plate with hands. Set aside in refrigerator or freezer, if preferred.

4. For *Lemon Curd Filling*, zest 1 lemon, then juice all lemons into clean food processor or high-speed blender. Add soaked cashews, soaked dates or honey, salt, and vanilla and turmeric (optional). Process until smooth, about 2 minutes. Add enough soaking liquid or water to reach desired consistency. Mixture should be smooth, but not too runny.

5. Pour *Lemon Curd Filling* into *Crust* and smooth with spatula or back of a spoon. Tp pie with fresh blueberries.

6. Refrigerate at least 1 hour, until set. Slice and serve chilled

Easy Apricot Pie

Prep Time: 10 minutes*

Servings: 8

INGREDIENTS

Crust

1 cup raw cashews

1 cup raw macadamia nuts (or raw brazil nuts)

1/3 cup flaked or shredded coconut

1 cup dried pitted dates

1/2 teaspoon vanilla

Apricot Filling

3 cups dried apricots

1/2 lemon

Water

INSTRUCTIONS

1. *For *Apricot Filling*, soak 2 1/2 cups apricots in enough water to cover for 2 hours. Drain, reserving soaking liquid.

2. For *Crust*, place all ingredients in food processor or high-speed blender. Process until well ground and mixture sticks together, about 2 minutes.

3. Press *Crust* firmly into pie plate, cake pan or baking dish with hands. Set aside in refrigerator or freezer, if preferred.

4. For *Apricot Filling*, zest then juice lemon into clean food processor or high-speed blender. Add soaked apricots and process until

smooth, about 1 - 2 minutes. Add enough soaking liquid to reach desired consistency. Mixture should be thick and smooth, but not runny.

5. Pour *Apricot Filling* into *Crust* and smooth with spatula or back of a spoon. Chop remaining unsoaked apricots and sprinkle over pie.

6. Slice and serve immediately. Or refrigerate at least 1 hour and serve chilled.

Blue Ribbon Apple Pie

Prep Time: 25 minutes*

Servings: 8

INGREDIENTS

Topping

1/2 cup raw pecans

1/2 cup raw walnuts

1/2 cup raw almonds

Crust

1 cup raw almonds

1 cup raw pecans

1 cup raw walnuts

1 1/2 cups dried pitted dates

1 teaspoon vanilla

1/2 teaspoon ground cinnamon

1/2 teaspoon Celtic sea salt

Apple Filling

3 apples

1/4 - 1/3 cup dried pitted dates

1/2 lemon

2 tablespoons flax seeds

1 teaspoon vanilla

1 teaspoon ground cinnamon

1/2 teaspoon Celtic sea salt

Water

INSTRUCTIONS

1. *For *Apple Filling*, soak dates in enough water to cover for 1 hour, then drain.

2. For *Topping*, add nuts to food processor or high-speed blender. Pulse until finely chopped. Set aside.

3. For *Crust*, place all ingredients in food processor or high-speed blender. Process until well ground and mixture sticks together, about 2 - 3 minutes.

4. Press *Crust* firmly into pie plate, cake pan or baking dish with hands. Set aside in refrigerator or freezer, if preferred.

5. For *Apple Filling*, add flax to clean food processor or high-speed blender and process until finely ground, about 1 minute.

6. Peel and core apples, then roughly chop. Juice lemon and add to processor with 1/3 of apples, soaked dates, vanilla and salt. Process until smooth, about 2 minutes.

7. Add 1/2 of remaining apples and process until finely chopped, but still chunky. Add remaining apples and pulse until roughly chopped. Set aside 15 minutes.

8. Pour *Apple Filling* into *Crust* and smooth with spatula or back of a spoon. Evenly sprinkle *Topping* over pie to create top crust.

9. Slice and serve immediately. Or refrigerate at least 1 hour and serve chilled.

Perfect Peach Pie

Prep Time: 10 minutes*

Servings: 8

INGREDIENTS

Crust

1 cup raw pecans

1 cup raw walnuts

1 cup dried pitted dates

1/2 teaspoon vanilla

1/2 teaspoon ground cinnamon

1/4 teaspoon Celtic sea salt

Peach Filling

4 ripe peaches (or nectarines)

1 teaspoon ground cinnamon

1/2 teaspoon ground nutmeg

1/4 teaspoon vanilla

1/4 teaspoon ground ginger (optional)

INSTRUCTIONS

1. For *Crust*, place all ingredients in food processor or high-speed blender. Process until well ground and mixture sticks together, about 2 minutes.

2. Press *Crust* firmly into pie plate, cake pan or baking dish with hands. Set aside in refrigerator or freezer, if preferred.

3. For *Peach Filling*, cut peaches in half and remove pit. Thinly slice and add to large mixing bowl. Sprinkle on spices and salt. Gently toss to coat evenly.
4. Pour *Peach Filling* and press into *Crust*.
5. Slice and serve immediately. Or refrigerate at least 1 hour and serve chilled.

1st Prize Cherry Pie

Prep Time: 15 minutes*

Servings: 8

INGREDIENTS

Crust

1 1/2 cups raw hazelnuts (or macadamia nuts)

1 cup raw almonds

1/4 cup dried pitted dates

1 teaspoon ground cinnamon

Blueberry Filling

4 cups pitted cherries (fresh or thawed)

1/4 cup raw coconut oil (or raw coconut or cacao butter, melted)

1/4 dried pitted dates

1/2 teaspoon vanilla

Pinch Celtic sea salt

INSTRUCTIONS

1. *For *Crust*, soak dates in enough water to cover for 1 hour, then drain.

2. Add nuts to food processor or high-speed blender and process until coarsely ground, about 1 minute. Add dates and cinnamon and process until mixture is well ground and sticks together, about 1 minute.

3. Press *Crust* firmly into pie plate, cake pan or baking dish with hands. Set aside in refrigerator or freezer, if preferred.

4. *For *Cherry Filling*, pit whole cherries, if using.

5. Add 1/3 of pitted cherries to clean food processor or high-speed blender with coconut oil or butter, dates, vanilla and salt. Process until smooth, about 1 - 2 minutes.

6. Add 1/2 of remaining cherries to processor and pulse to roughly chop.

7. Pour *Cherry Filling* into *Crust* and smooth with spatula or back of a spoon. Roughly chop or halve remaining cherries. Sprinkle remaining cherries over pie.

8. *Refrigerate at least 1 hour, until set. Slice and serve chilled. Or allow to warm slightly and serve.

Fruity Blueberry Pie

Prep Time: 15 minutes*

Servings: 8

INGREDIENTS

Crust

1 cup raw almonds (or raw pecans)

1 cup dried pitted dates

1 1/2 cups flaked or shredded coconut

1/2 lemon

1 teaspoon vanilla

Pinch Celtic sea salt

Blueberry Filling

2 cups blueberries (fresh or thawed)

1/2 cup raw coconut oil (or raw coconut or cacao butter, melted)

1/4 cup cashew butter(or 1/2 cup raw cashews)

1/4 - 1/3 cup dried pitted dates

1/2 lemon

1 teaspoon vanilla

1/4 teaspoon Celtic sea salt

INSTRUCTIONS

1. For *Crust*, add almonds to food processor or high-speed blender and process until finely ground, about 2 minutes. Zest *then* juice lemon in to processer with remaining *Crust* ingredients. Process until mixture is well ground and sticks together, about 2 minutes.

2. Press *Crust* firmly into pie plate, cake pan or baking dish with hands. Set aside in refrigerator or freezer, if preferred.

3. For *Blueberry Filling*, zest *then* juice lemon into clean food processor or high-speed blender. Add raw cashews and blend until smooth, if using.

4. Or add cashew butter, dates, and coconut oil or butter to processor. Process until smooth, about 1 - 2 minutes.

5. Add 1 1/2 cups blueberries, vanilla and salt to processor. Process until thick smooth mixture forms, about 1 minute.

6. Pour *Blueberry Filling* into *Crust* and smooth with spatula or back of a spoon. Sprinkle remaining blueberries over pie.

7. Slice and serve immediately. Or refrigerate at least 1 hour and serve chilled.

Refrigerator Carrot Cake

Prep Time: 10 minutes*

Servings: 8

INGREDIENTS

Carrot Cake

2 - 3 large carrots

2 cups raw walnuts

1/2 cup raisins (or dried apricots)

1/2 cup flaked or shredded coconut

2 tablespoons raw pumpkin seeds

1/4 cup raw honey (or dried pitted dates)

1 teaspoon vanilla

1 teaspoon ground cinnamon

1/4teaspoon ground nutmeg

1/4 teaspoon ground ginger (optional)

Cashew Cream Icing

1 cup raw cashews

1/2 large lemon

2 tablespoons raw honey (or dried pitted dates)

1 teaspoon vanilla

Water

INSTRUCTIONS

1. *For *Cashew Cream Icing*, separately soak cashews and dates (if using) in enough water to cover for 2 hours. Drain dates. Drain and rinse cashews.

2. For *Carrot Cake*, add carrots to food processor or high-speed blender and pulse to roughly chop. Add all *Carrot Cake* ingredients and process until coarsely ground but still slightly chunky, about 1 minute.

3. Transfer mixture to cake or baking pan and press firmly with hands.

4. For *Cashew Cream Icing*, juice lemon and add to clean food processor or high-speed blender with soaked cashews, soaked dates or honey, and vanilla. Process until smooth, about 2 minutes. Add enough date soaking liquid or water to reach desired consistency.

5. Spread *Cashew Cream Icing* over *Carrot Cake* and place in refrigerator at least 2 hours.

6. Slice and serve chilled. Or allow to warm slightly and serve.

Tasty Chocolate Cake

Prep Time: 10 minutes*

Servings: 8

INGREDIENTS

Chocolate Cake

1 1/2 cups raw pecans

1 1/2 cups raw walnuts

1 1/2 cups dried pitted dates

1 1/2 cups raisins (or dried apricots or other dried fruit)

1/3 cup raw cocoa powder

2 teaspoons vanilla

Chocolate Icing

1 cup raw cashews

4 tablespoons raw honey (or dried pitted dates)

2 tablespoons raw cocoa powder

1/2 teaspoon vanilla

Water

INSTRUCTIONS

1. *For *Chocolate Icing*, separately soak cashews and dates (if using) in enough water to cover for 2 hours. Drain dates. Drain and rinse cashews.

2. For *Chocolate Cake*, add pecans and walnuts to food processor or high-speed blender. Process until coarsely ground, about 1 minute.

3. Add dates and process until finely ground, about 1 minute. Repeat with raisins, then cocoa and vanilla.

4. Process all ingredients until dough comes together. Transfer mixture to cake or baking pan and press firmly with hands.

5. For *Chocolate Icing*, add soaked cashews, soaked dates or honey, cocoa and vanilla to clean food processor or high-speed blender. Process until smooth, about 2 minutes. Add enough date soaking liquid or water to reach desired consistency.

6. Pour *Chocolate Icing* over *Chocolate Cake* and smooth with spatula or back of a spoon.

7. Refrigerate at least 1 hour, until cake is firm. Slice and serve chilled. Or allow to warm slightly and serve.

New Country Red Velvet Cake

Prep Time: 15 minutes*

Servings: 8

INGREDIENTS

Red Velvet Cake

1 cup raw cashews

1 cup flaked or shredded coconut

1 cup dried pitted dates

4 beets (about 2 cups shredded)

1 large apple (or pear)

2 tablespoons raw coconut oil (or raw coconut or cacao butter, melted)

1 teaspoon vanilla

1/4 teaspoon Celtic sea salt

Cashew Frosting

1 cup raw cashews

1/3 cup dried pitted dates

2 tablespoons raw coconut oil (or raw coconut or cacao butter, melted)

1 teaspoon vanilla

Pinch Celtic sea salt

Water

INSTRUCTIONS

1. *For *Red Velvet Cake* and *Cashew Frosting*, separately soak cashews and dates in enough water to cover for 2 hours. Drain dates. Drain and rinse cashews.

2. For *Red Velvet Cake*, scrub and rinse beets. Remove roots and stems, and add to food processor or high-speed blender. Process to finely chop, about 2 minutes.

3. Peel and core apple. Add to processor and process to coarsely grind, about 1 minute.

4. Add coconut, soaked cashews and dates, coconut oil or butter, vanilla and salt. Process until mixture is finely ground and fairly smooth, up to 5 minutes.

5. Transfer mixture to cake or baking pan and press firmly with hands. Set aside in freezer.

6. For *Cashew Frosting*, add soaked cashews and dates, coconut oil or butter, vanilla and salt to clean food processor or high-speed blender. Process until smooth, about 2 minutes. Add enough date soaking liquid or water to reach desired consistency.

7. Spread *Cashew Frosting* over *Red Velvet Cake.*

8. Refrigerate or freeze at least 1 hour. Slice and serve chilled. Or allow to warm slightly and serve.

9. Store leftovers in freezer.

Sweet Treat Banana Bread

Prep Time: 10 minutes*

Dehydrating Time: 14 - 16 hours

Servings: 8

INGREDIENTS

Banana Bread

1 cup raw almonds

2 ripe bananas

2 sweet apples

2 carrots

1/2 cup flax meal (or flax seeds)

1/4 cup dried pitted dates

1/4 cup chopped walnuts

INSTRUCTIONS

1. Add whole flax to food processor or high-speed blender, if using. Process until finely ground, about 2 minutes.

2. Transfer flax meal to medium mixing bowl.

3. Add almonds to processor and process until finely ground, about 2 minutes. Add to flax.

4. Peel and core apples. Peel bananas. Roughly chop and add to processor. Process until puréed, about 2 minutes. Add to almond and flax meal.

5. Add carrots and dates to processor. Process until puréed, about 2 - 3 minutes. Add enough water to reached desired consistency, if necessary.

6. Add carrot and date purée to mixing bowl with walnuts. Mix to combine. Mixture should stick together. Add flax meal and/or water to reach desired consistency, if necessary.

7. Line dehydrator tray with dehydrator or parchment sheet.

8. Form mixture into loaves and place on lined dehydrator tray. Dehydrate at 118 degrees F for 14 - 16 hours. Until the outside is firm to the touch but the inside is still moist.

9. Remove from dehydrator and slice. Transfer to serving dish serve immediately. Or store in airtight container.

Scrumptious Coconut Macaroons

Prep Time: 15 minutes

Dehydrating Time: 24 hours

Servings: 12

INGREDIENTS

2 1/2 cups flaked or shredded coconut

1/3 cup dried pitted dates

1/3 cup water

1/2 teaspoon vanilla

Pinch Celtic sea salt

INSTRUCTIONS

1. Add 1 1/4 cups coconut to food processor or high-speed blender. Process until smooth and creamy, up to 5 minutes. Scrape down sides of bowl as necessary.

2. Add dates, water, vanilla and salt to processor. Process until smooth, about 2 minutes.

3. Transfer mixture to medium mixing bowl. Add remaining coconut and mix until well combined.

4. Line dehydrator tray with dehydrator or parchment sheets.

5. Use scoop or tablespoon to drop cookies onto lined dehydrator trays. Dehydrate at 118 degrees F for about 24 hours. Until the outside is dry to the touch but the inside is still moist.

6. Remove from dehydrator and transfer to serving dish. Serve immediately. Or store in airtight container.

Dunkable Chocolate Chunk Cookies

Prep Time: 20 minutes*

Dehydrating Time: 6 - 12 hours

Servings: 12

INGREDIENTS

2 cups raw cashew flour (or 3 cups raw cashews)

1 cup almond butter (or 1 1/2 cups raw almonds)

2 tablespoons raw coconut oil (or raw coconut or cacao butter, melted)

1 tablespoon flax meal

3/4 cup dried pitted dates

2 teaspoons vanilla

1 teaspoon Celtic sea salt

1 cup raw chocolate chips (or cacao nibs or raw chocolate bark)

Water

INSTRUCTIONS

1. *Soak dates in enough water to cover for at least 6 hours, or overnight in refrigerator. Drain, reserving soaking liquid.

2. Add cashews to food processor or high-speed blender. Process until finely ground, about 2 minutes. Transfer cashew flour to medium mixing bowl.

3. Add almonds (if using) to processor and process until smooth and creamy, up to 8 minutes. Scrape down as necessary.

4. Add dates, coconut oil or butter, flax, vanilla and salt to almond butter in processor. Process until smooth, about 1 - 2 minutes. Transfer mixture to mixing bowl.

5. Chop raw chocolate bark, if using. Add cacao nibs or raw chocolate and mix well to combine. Add date soaking liquid to reach desired consistency. Dough should be moist and stick together.
6. Line dehydrator trays with dehydrator or parchment sheets.
7. Form mixture into balls and place on dehydrator or parchment sheets. Press to flatten.
8. Place in dehydrator and dehydrate at 118 degrees F for about 6 - 12 hours, depending on desired crispiness. Outside should be firm while inside is still moist.
9. Remove from dehydrator and transfer to serving dish. Serve immediately. Or store in airtight container.

Dehydrated Almond Biscotti

Prep Time: 10 minutes*

Dehydrating Time: 12 - 24 hours

Servings: 12

INGREDIENTS

1 1/2 cups raw almond flour

2 cups raw almonds

1 cup flaked or shredded coconut

1/2 cup raw honey (or dried pitted dates)

1/2 cup dried apricots or golden raisins (optional)

1 teaspoon vanilla

1/4 teaspoon Celtic sea salt

Water

INSTRUCTIONS

1. *Soak dates in enough water to cover overnight in refrigerator, if using. Drain, reserving soaking liquid.

2. Add 1 1/2 cups almonds to food processor or high-speed blender. Process until finely ground, about 2 minutes.

3. Add coconut to processor and process until finely ground, about 1 minute.

4. Add soaked dates or honey, vanilla, salt, and apricots or raisins (optional) to processor. Process until well ground, about 1 - 2 minutes. Transfer mixture to mixing bowl.

5. Add almond flour and remaining 1/2 cup raw almonds. Mix well to combine. Add date soaking liquid to reach desired consistency. Dough should be moist and stick together.
6. Line dehydrator trays with dehydrator or parchment sheets.
7. Form mixture into loaves and place on dehydrator or parchment sheets.
8. Place in dehydrator and dehydrate at 118 degrees F for about 8 hours.
9. Remove from dehydrator and cut into 3/4 inch slices. Turn slices on sides and place directly on dehydrator tray. Continue dehydrating 4 - 16 hours, depending on desired crispiness.
10. Remove from dehydrator and transfer to serving dish. Serve immediately. Or store in airtight container.

Ginger Punch Pudding

Prep Time: 20 minutes*

Servings: 2

INGREDIENTS

1 young coconut (about 1 cup coconut meat and 1 cup coconut water)

2 - 4 tablespoons raw honey (or pitted dates)

1 1/2 inch piece fresh ginger

1/2 teaspoon ground ginger

1 teaspoon vanilla

Water (optional)

INSTRUCTIONS

1. * Soak dates in enough water to cover for at least 4 hours, or overnight in refrigerator (if using). Drain.

2. Remove flesh from fresh coconut and add to high-speed blender with 1 cup coconut water. Process until well blended and fairly smooth, about 1 - 2 minutes.

3. Peel ginger and grate into processor. Add vanilla, ground ginger, and honey or dates. Process until smooth, about 1 minute.

4. Transfer to serving dish and serve immediately or refrigerate at least 20 minutes and serve chilled.

Creamy Strawberry Ice Cream

Prep Time: 30 minutes

Servings: 4

INGREDIENTS

2 coconuts (or 1 cup flaked coconut)

2 tablespoons raw honey (or dried pitted dates)

2 cup strawberries (fresh or thawed)

1/2 teaspoon vanilla

Water

INSTRUCTIONS

1. *Freeze ice cream maker canister for overnight.
2. *Soak flaked coconut and dates in 2 cups water overnight in refrigerator, if using.
3. Add soaked coconut and dates, plus soaking liquid to high-speed blender. Process until well blended and fairly smooth, about 1 - 2 minutes.
4. Or remove flesh from fresh coconuts and add to high-speed blender with 2 cups water. Process until well blended and fairly smooth, about 1 - 2 minutes.
5. Strain mixture through nut milk bag, cheesecloth or strainer back into blender.
6. Reserve pulp and set aside to dry and dehydrate, then use as coconut flour.

7. Remove stems from strawberries, then cut in half. Add to blender with honey or dates, and vanilla. Process until smooth, about 1 minute.
8. Turn on ice cream maker. Slowly pour mixture into running ice cream maker. Let machine run until ice cream forms, about 20 minutes.
9. Transfer to serving dish and serve immediately. Or store in airtight container in freezer.

Tropical Sorbet

Prep Time: 30 minutes

Servings: 4

INGREDIENTS

2 coconuts (or 1 cup flaked coconut)

3 ripe mangos

1 orange

INSTRUCTIONS

1. *Freeze ice cream maker canister overnight.
2. *Soak flaked coconut in 2 cups water overnight in refrigerator, if using.
3. Add soaked coconut and soaking liquid to high-speed blender. Process until well blended and fairly smooth, about 1 - 2 minutes.
4. Or remove flesh from fresh coconuts and add to high-speed blender with 2 cups water. Process until well blended and fairly smooth, about 1 - 2 minutes.
5. Strain mixture through nut milk bag, cheesecloth or strainer back into blender.
6. Reserve pulp and set aside to dry and dehydrate, then use as coconut flour.
7. Cut mangos in half and remove peel. Roughly chop and add to blender. Zest *then* juice orange. Add to processor and process until smooth, about 1 minute.

8. Turn on ice cream maker. Slowly pour mixture into running ice cream maker. Let machine run until ice cream forms, about 20 minutes.

9. Transfer to serving dish and serve immediately. Or store in airtight container in freezer.

Smoothies Recipes

Homemade Almond Milk

Prep Time: 5 minutes*

Servings: 2

INGREDIENTS

1 cup raw almonds

4 cups water

INSTRUCTIONS

1. *Soak almonds in 1 cup water at least 6 hours, or overnight.
2. Drain soaked almonds and add to high-speed blender with 3 cups water. Process until well blended and almost smooth, about 1- 2 minutes.
3. Strain mixture through nut milk bag, cheesecloth or strainer into container.
4. Keep refrigerated up to 4 days. If milk separates, mix before use.

Homemade Coconut Milk

Prep Time: 10 minutes

Servings: 2

INGREDIENTS

2 mature coconuts

3 cups water

INSTRUCTIONS

1. Remove flesh from coconuts and add to high-speed blender with 3 cups water. Process until well blended and fairly smooth, about 1- 2 minutes.

2. Strain mixture through nut milk bag, cheesecloth or strainer into container.

3. Reserve pulp and set aside to dry and dehydrate, then use as coconut flour.

4. Keep refrigerated up to 4 days. If milk separates, mix before use.

NOTE: Blend additional coconut flesh with prepared coconut milk and strain for thicker coconut milk. Continue blending thickened coconut milk with additional coconut flesh until coconut cream forms. Or set thickened milk aside in refrigerator and allow fat to separate for coconut cream.

Shredded Coconut Milk

Prep Time: 5 minutes*

Servings: 2

INGREDIENTS

2 cups dried coconut (unsweetened shreds or flakes)

4 cups of water

INSTRUCTIONS

1. *Soak dried coconut in 3 cups water at least 6 hours, or overnight in refrigerator.
2. Add soaked coconut and liquid to high-speed blender. Process until well blended and fairly smooth, about 1- 2 minutes. Add extra water for thinner consistency.
3. Strain mixture through nut milk bag, cheesecloth or strainer into container.
4. Reserve pulp and set aside to dry and dehydrate, then use as coconut flour.
5. Keep refrigerated up to 4 days. If milk separates, mix before use.

NOTE: Increase coconut and decrease water for thicker coconut milk. Set thickened milk aside in refrigerator and allow fat to separate for coconut cream.

Green Supreme Smoothie

Prep Time: 5 minutes*

Servings: 1

INGREDIENTS

1 cup chopped kale

1/2 cup watercress

1 banana (frozen chunks)

1 green apple

1/2 avocado

1 1/2 cups nut milk (or kefir)

2 - 4 tablespoons sweetener** (optional)

INSTRUCTIONS

1. *Peel banana, then chop and freeze.
2. Remove any stems and ribs from kale. Peel apple if preferred, then core and dice.
3. Slice avocado in half and scoop flesh of pitted half into high-speed blender. Add remaining ingredients and process until smooth, about 1 - 2 minutes.
4. Pour into large glass and serve immediately.

Stevia, dried dates or raw honey

Sweet Envy Green Smoothie

Prep Time: 5 minutes

Servings: 1

INGREDIENTS

1 cup spinach

1 small zucchini (or 1/2 large)

2 celery stalks

1 cup green grapes

1 1/4 cups nut milk

2 - 4 tablespoons sweetener* (optional)

INSTRUCTIONS

1. Peel zucchini if preferred, then chop. Chop celery stalks.
2. Add all ingredients to high-speed blender. Process until smooth, about 1 - 2 minutes.
3. Pour into large glass and serve immediately.

*Stevia, dried dates or raw honey

Perfect Pear Smoothie

Prep Time: 5 minutes*

Servings: 1

INGREDIENTS

2 ripe pears

1 banana (frozen chunks)

1 1/4 cups nut milk

1/2 teaspoon ground cinnamon

1/4 teaspoon ground nutmeg

1/4 teaspoon vanilla

INSTRUCTIONS

1. *Peel banana, then cut into chucks and freeze.
2. Stem and seed pears, then cut into quarters.
3. Add all ingredients to high-speed blender. Process until smooth, about 1 minute.
4. Pour into large glass and serve immediately.

Red Rave Smoothie

Prep Time: 5 minutes

Servings: 1

INGREDIENTS

1 cup strawberries (frozen halves)

1/2 cup red raspberries

1/2 cup pitted cherries

1 cup nut milk

1 tablespoon chia or flax seed (optional)

INSTRUCTIONS

1. *Remove stems from strawberries, then cut in half and freeze.
2. Pit cherries, if fresh.
3. Add frozen strawberries and nut milk to high speed blender. Pulse to break down frozen strawberries.
4. Add remaining ingredients and process until smooth, about 1 minute.
5. Pour into large glass and serve immediately.

Strawberry Banana Blend

Prep Time: 5 minutes*

Servings: 1

INGREDIENTS

1 banana (frozen chunks)

1 cup strawberries (frozen halves)

1 1/2 cup nut milk

1/4 teaspoon vanilla

INSTRUCTIONS

1. *Peel banana, then cut into chucks and freeze. Remove stems from strawberries, cut in half and freeze.
2. Add all ingredients to high-speed blender. Process until smooth, about 1- 2 minutes.
3. Pour into large glass and serve immediately.

Tropical Colada Mombata

Prep Time: 5 minutes*

Servings: 1

INSTRUCTIONS

1 small banana (frozen chunks)

1 cup pineapple (frozen chunks)

1 1/2 cups coconut milk

2 tablespoons flaked coconut (or 1/4 cup fresh coconut)

DIRECTIONS

1. *Peel banana, then cut into chucks and freeze. Peel pineapple, then cut into chunks and freeze.
2. Add all ingredients to high-speed blender. Process until smooth, about 1- 2 minutes.
3. Pour into large glass and serve immediately.

Kiwi Strawberry Smoothie

Prep Time: 5 minutes*

Servings: 1

INGREDIENTS

1 cup strawberries (frozen halves)

2 kiwis

1 cup nut milk

1/2 cup orange juice (about 2 oranges)

1 tablespoon chia or flax seed (optional)

INSTRUCTIONS

1. *Remove stems from strawberries, cut in half and freeze.
2. Peel kiwi and cut into quarters. Juice oranges.
3. Add all ingredients to high-speed blender. Process until smooth, about 1- 2 minutes.
4. Pour into large glass and serve immediately.

Peter Rabbit Carrot Crush

Prep Time: 10 minutes*

Servings: 1

INGREDIENTS

1 small banana (frozen chunks)

1/2 cup pineapple (frozen chunks)

2 large carrots

Small piece ginger root

1/2 cup orange juice (about 2 oranges)

1 cup nut milk

1/2 teaspoon ground cinnamon

1 cage-free egg (optional)

INSTRUCTIONS

1. *Peel banana, then cut into chucks and freeze. Peel pineapple, then cut into chunks and freeze.
2. Juice carrots, oranges and ginger root.
3. Add all ingredients to high-speed blender. Process until smooth, about 1- 2 minutes.
4. Pour into large glass and serve immediately.

Chocolate Banana Shake

Prep Time: 5 minutes

Servings: 1

INGREDIENTS

1 large banana (or 2 small)

2 tablespoons raw cocoa powder

1 cup nut milk

1/2 cup ice

2 - 4 tablespoons sweetener* (optional)

INSTRUCTIONS

1. Peel and chop banana.
2. Add ice and nut milk to high-speed blender. Pulse to crush ice.
3. Add remaining ingredients and process until smooth, about 1- 2 minutes.
4. Pour into large glass and serve immediately.

Stevia, dried dates or raw honey

Cucumber Melon Slushy

Prep Time: 5 minutes*

Servings: 2

INGREDIENTS

1 small cucumber

1 cup watermelon (chunks)

1 cup honeydew melon (frozen chunks)

1 cup coconut milk

2 - 4 tablespoons sweetener** (optional)

INSTRUCTIONS

1. * Cut honeydew flesh away from peel, then cut into chunks and freeze.
2. Peel cucumber and remove seeds, then cut into chunks. Cut watermelon flesh away from rind, then remove seeds and cut into chunks.
3. Add all ingredients to high-speed blender. Process until smooth, about 1 minute.
4. Pour into large glasses and serve immediately.

**Stevia, dried dates or raw honey*

Sweet Strawberry Slushy

Prep Time: 5 minutes*

Servings: 1

INGREDIENTS

1 cup strawberries

1 cup strawberries (frozen halves)

2 cups coconut milk

1/2 teaspoon vanilla

2 tablespoons chia or flax seed (optional)

INSTRUCTIONS

1. * Remove stems from 1 cup strawberries, then cut in half and freeze.
2. Remove stems from 1 cup fresh strawberries.
3. Add frozen strawberries and coconut milk to high-speed blender. Pulse to break down frozen strawberries.
4. Add remaining ingredients and process until smooth, about 1- 2 minutes.
5. Pour into large glass and serve immediately.

Sweet Berry Bliss

Prep Time: 5 minutes*

Servings: 1

INGREDIENTS

1 banana (frozen chunks)

1/2 cup strawberries (frozen halves)

1/4 cup blueberries

1/4 cup blackberries

1 1/2 cups nut milk

1/2 teaspoon vanilla

2 tablespoons chia or flax seed (optional)

INSTRUCTIONS

1. *Peel banana, then cut into chucks and freeze. Remove stems from strawberries, then cut in half and freeze.
2. Add all ingredients to high-speed blender. Process until smooth, about 1 - 2 minutes.
3. Pour into large glass and serve immediately.

Indigo Blue Berry Blend

Prep Time: 5 minutes

Servings: 1

INGREDIENTS

1 cup blueberries (frozen)

1/4 cup black raspberries

1/4 cup blackberries

1/4 cup pitted black cherries

1 /2 cups nut milk

1/2 teaspoon vanilla

2 tablespoons chia or flax seed (optional)

INSTRUCTIONS

1. *Freeze blueberries.
2. Add alls ingredients to high-speed blender. Process until smooth, about 1 minute.
3. Pour into large glass and serve immediately.

Nutty Buddy Banana Smoothie

Prep Time: 5 minutes*

Servings: 1

INGREDIENTS

1 banana (frozen chunks)

1/4 cup raw almond butter (or 1/2 cup raw almonds)

1 cup nut milk

2 - 4 tablespoons sweetener**

INSTRUCTIONS

1. *Peel banana, then cut into chucks and freeze.
2. Add raw almonds to food processor or high speed blender and process until smooth, about 3 minutes. Or use prepared raw almond butter.
3. Add all ingredients to high-speed blender. Process until smooth, about 1 - 2 minutes.
4. Pour into large glass and serve immediately.

**Stevia, dried dates or raw honey

Bright & Early Orange Whirl

Prep Time: 5 minutes

Servings: 1

INGREDIENTS

1 1/2 cups orange or tangerine juice (about 6 oranges or 10 tangerines)

1/2 cup coconut cream (or thick coconut milk)

2/3 cup ice

1 cage-free egg (optional)

2 tablespoons sweetener* (optional)

INSTRUCTIONS

1. Juice oranges.
2. Add ice and orange juice to high-speed blender. Pulse to crush ice.
3. Add remaining ingredients and process until smooth, about 1 minute.
4. Pour into large glass and serve immediately.

*Stevia, dried dates or raw honey

Sweet Mango Swirl

Prep Time: 5 minutes

Servings: 1

INGREDIENTS

1 ripe mango

1 cup coconut milk

1/2 cup ice

1 cage-free egg (optional)

2 - 4 tablespoons sweetener* (optional)

INSTRUCTIONS

1. Cut flesh of mango from pit. Remove peel and cut into chunks.
2. Add ice and coconut milk to high-speed blender. Pulse to crush ice.
3. Add remaining ingredients and process until smooth, about 1 minute.
4. Pour into large glass and serve immediately.

Stevia, dried dates or raw honey

Strawberry Orange Smoothie

Prep Time: 5 minutes*

Servings: 1

INGREDIENTS

1 cup strawberries

1/2 cup strawberries (frozen halves)

1 cup orange juice (about 4 oranges)

1/2 cup thick coconut milk (or kefir)

2 tablespoons chia or flax seed (optional)

INSTRUCTIONS

1. *Remove stems from 1/2 cup strawberries, then cut in half and freeze.
2. Remove stem from fresh strawberries. Juice oranges
3. Add frozen strawberries and orange juice to high-speed blender. Pulse to break down frozen strawberries.
4. Add remaining ingredients and process until smooth, about 1 minute.
5. Pour into large glass and serve immediately.

Sweet Avocado Swirl

Prep Time: 5 minutes

Servings: 1

INGREDIENTS

1 ripe avocado

1 cup coconut milk (or kefir)

1/3 cup ice

1/2 teaspoon vanilla

2 - 4 tablespoons sweetener*

2 tablespoons raw cocoa powder (optional)

INSTRUCTIONS

1. Add ice and coconut milk to high-speed blender. Pulse to crush ice.

2. Slice avocado in half and remove pit. Scoop into high-speed blender.

3. Add remaining ingredients and process until smooth, about 1 minute.

4. Pour into large glass and serve immediately.

*Stevia, dried dates or raw honey

Watermelon Cooler Crush

Prep Time: 5 minutes*

Servings: 1

INGREDIENTS

2 cups watermelon (chunks)

1/2 cup strawberries (frozen halves)

2 limes

1/2 cup thick coconut milk

2 - 4 tablespoons sweetener**

INSTRUCTIONS

1. *Remove stems from strawberries, then cut in halve and freeze.
2. Cut watermelon flesh away from rind and cut into chunks. Juice limes.
3. Add frozen strawberries, lime juice and nut milk to high-speed blender. Pulse to break down frozen strawberries.
4. Add all ingredients and to high-speed blender. process until smooth, about 1 minute.
5. Pour into large glass and serve immediately.

**Stevia, dried dates or raw honey

Bananarama Blend

Prep Time: 5 minutes*

Servings: 1

INGREDIENTS

1 banana (frozen chunks)

1 plum

1/4 cup pitted prunes

1 cup nut milk

1/2 cup orange juice (about 2 oranges)

1 cage-free egg (optional)

INSTRUCTIONS

1. *Peel banana, then cut into chucks and freeze.
2. Cut plum in half and remove pit, then quarter. Juice oranges.
3. Add all ingredients to high-speed blender. Process until smooth, about 1 - 2 minutes.
4. Pour into large glass and serve immediately.

Peach Relief Smoothie

Prep Time: 5 minutes

Servings: 1

INGREDIENTS

1 ripe peach or nectarine (frozen chunks)

2 fresh apricots (or 1/4 cup dried)

1/2 cup nut milk (or kefir)

1/2 cup fresh orange juice (about 2 oranges)

1 cage-free egg (optional)

INSTRUCTIONS

1. *Cut peach in half and remove pit, then cut into chucks and freeze.
2. Cut fresh apricots in half and remove pits, then cut into chucks, if using. Juice oranges.
3. Add all ingredients to high-speed blender. Process until smooth, about 1 minute.
4. Pour into large glass and serve immediately.

Morning Mellow Melon

Prep Time: 5 minutes*

Servings: 1

INGREDIENTS

1 cup honeydew melon (frozen chunks)

1 cup cantaloupe (chunks)

1 grapefruit (about 2/3 cup juice)

2/3 cup thick coconut milk

2 - 4 tablespoons sweetener**

INSTRUCTIONS

1. *Cut honeydew melon flesh away from rind, then cut into chunks and freeze.
2. Cut cantaloupe flesh away from rind, then cut into chunks. Juice grapefruit.
3. Add frozen honeydew chunks and grapefruit juice to high-speed blender. Pulse to break down frozen honeydew.
4. Add remaining ingredients and process until smooth, about 1 minute.
5. Pour into large glass and serve immediately.

**Stevia, dried dates or raw honey*

Guava Pop Smoothie

Prep Time: 5 minutes

Servings: 1

INGREDIENTS

1 mango (frozen chunks)

1/2 cup papaya (chunks)

1 ripe guava

2 limes

1 cup coconut milk

INSTRUCTIONS

1. *Cut mango flesh away from pit and peel. Then dice into small chunks and freeze.
2. Peel papaya and remove seeds, then cut into chunks. Peel guava if preferred, then cut in half. Juice limes.
3. Add coconut milk and guava to high-speed blender. Process until smooth. Strain out seeds, reserving liquid.
4. Add strained guava mixture back to high-speed blender with frozen mango chunks. Pulse to break down frozen mango.
5. Add remaining ingredients and process until smooth, about 1 minute.
6. Pour into large glass and serve immediately.

Lemon Freeze

Prep Time: 5 minutes

Servings: 1

INGREDIENTS

1/2 cup fresh lemon juice (about 3 lemons)

1/2 cup fresh orange juice (about 2 oranges)

1/2 cup coconut milk

1/2 cup ice

2 - 4 tablespoons sweetener*

INSTRUCTIONS

1. Juice lemons and oranges.
2. Add ice and coconut milk to high-speed blender. Pulse to crush ice.
3. Add remaining ingredients and process until smooth, about 1 minute.
4. Pour into large glass and serve immediately.

*Stevia, dried dates or raw honey

Mojito Cooler Crush

Prep Time: 5 minutes

Servings: 1

INGREDIENTS

1/2 cup lime juice (about 5 limes)

1 sprig fresh mint

1/2 cup thick coconut milk

2 tablespoons flaked coconut (or 1/4 cup fresh coconut)

1/2 cup ice

2 - 4 tablespoons sweetener*

1/2 teaspoon vanilla (optional)

INSTRUCTIONS

1. Remove mint leaves from stem. Juice limes.
2. Add ice and limes juice to high-speed blender. Pulse to crush ice.
3. Add remaining ingredients to high-speed blender and process until smooth, about 1 minute.
4. Pour into large glass and serve immediately.

*Stevia, dried dates or raw honey

On the Go Recipes

Lemon Energy Bars

Prep Time: 25 minutes

Servings: 6

INGREDIENTS

1 cup raw cashews

2 lemons

1/2 cup dried pineapple

1/2 cup flaked or shredded coconut

1/4 cup dried apricots

1/4 teaspoon ground ginger

1/4 teaspoon vanilla

Pinch Celtic sea salt

1/3 cup warm water

INSTRUCTIONS

1. Zest *then* juice lemons into small mixing bowl. Reserve half of juice and zest.

2. Soak dried pineapple and apricots in warm water and juice and zest of 1 lemon for 5 - 10 minutes.

3. Line loaf pan with parchment paper.

4. Add cashews to food processor or high-speed blender. Drain fruit and add to processor with coconut, salt, spices, and lemon juice and zest. Process for about 1 minute, until fruit and nuts break down and mixture sticks together when pressed.

5. Transfer mixture to prepared loaf pan and press firmly into bottom with hands or spatula.

6. Place in refrigerator and chill for 10 minutes. Remove and cut into 6 bars.

7. Serve immediately. Or store refrigerated in airtight container up to 2 weeks.

Ginger Crisps

Prep Time: 5 minutes

Dehydrating Time: 4 - 8 hours

Servings: 12

INGREDIENTS

2 cups raw almond flour

1 1/2 cups dried pitted dates

4 inch piece fresh ginger

2 tablespoons raw coconut oil (or raw cacao or coconut butter)

2 tablespoons raw honey

2 teaspoons ground ginger

1 teaspoons ground cinnamon

1/2 teaspoon ground black pepper (or ground white pepper)

1/2 teaspoon vanilla

1/4 teaspoon Celtic sea salt

INSTRUCTIONS

1. Peel and grate ginger. Add to food processor or high-speed blender with almond flour, dates, oil or butter, honey, salt and spices . Process until mixture is well ground and comes together, about 2 minutes.
2. Line dehydrator trays with dehydrator or parchment sheets.
3. Form mixture into 12 - 24 balls and place on lined dehydrator trays. Press to flatten.
4. Place in dehydrator and dehydrate at 115 degrees F for 4 - 8 hours, until desired crispiness is reached.

5. Remove from dehydrator and transfer to serving dish. Serve immediately. Or store in airtight container.

Crisp Cocoa Wafers

Prep Time: 10 minutes*

Dehydrating Time: 8 - 16 hours

Servings: 12

INGREDIENTS

1/2 cup almonds

3/4 cups cashews

1/3 cup dates

1/4 cup raw cocoa powder

1 tablespoon raw oil (coconut, walnut, almond, sesame, etc.)

1 teaspoon vanilla

1/4 teaspoon Celtic sea salt

Water

INSTRUCTIONS

1. *Soak almonds in enough water to cover for at least 6 hours, or overnight in refrigerator. Drain and rinse. Soak cashews and dates in enough water to cover for at least 1 hour. Drain.

2. Add soaked almonds and cashews to food processor or high-speed blender. Process until finely ground, about 1 - 2 minutes.

3. Add dates, cocoa, oil, vanilla and salt to processor. Process until mixture is well combined and sticks together, about 1 - 2 minutes.

4. Line dehydrator trays with dehydrator or parchment sheets.

5. Form mixture into 12 balls and place on dehydrator or parchment sheets. Press to flatten.

6. Place in dehydrator and dehydrate at 115 degrees F for about 8 - 16 hours, depending on desired crispiness.

7. Remove from dehydrator and transfer to serving dish. Serve immediately. Or store in airtight container.

Good Morning Trail Mix

Prep Time: 5 minutes

Servings: 4

INGREDIENTS

1/2 cup raw almonds

1/2 cup raw pumpkin seeds

1/2 cup cashews

1/4 cup golden raisins

1/4 cup dried blueberries

1/4 cup dried strawberries

INSTRUCTIONS

1. Roughly chop dried strawberries. Add to medium mixing bowl with fruit and nuts. Mix to combine.
2. Transfer to serving dish and serve immediately. Or store in airtight container.

Preserved Beef Jerky

Prep Time: 10 minutes*

Dehydrating Time: 4 - 8 hours

Servings: 4

INGREDIENTS

4 oz grass-fed beef

2 tablespoons coconut aminos (or liquid aminos or tamari)

2 tablespoons lemon juice (or raw apple cider vinegar)

1 tablespoons Celtic sea salt

1/2 teaspoon ground ginger

1/2 teaspoon garlic powder

1/2 teaspoon onion powder

1/2 teaspoon smoked paprika

1/2 teaspoon cayenne pepper

INSTRUCTIONS

1. Prepare two parchment sheets. Lay one on cutting board.

2. Cut slice beef into 1/4 inch strips and lay in single layer on parchment. Pound with tenderizing side of kitchen mallet. Cover beef with second parchment sheet, then pound with flat side of tenderizing mallet to 1/8 inch thickness.

3. *Place beef strips in medium mixing bowl or shallow dish. Add coconut aminos, lemon juice, salt and spices. Mix well to coat. Cover and place in refrigerator for 8 hours, or overnight.

4. Remove beef from refrigerator and lay in single layer on dehydrator trays. Place in dehydrator and dehydrate at 120 degrees F for 4 - 8 hours.

5. After 4 hours dehydrating time, remove trays from dehydrator and test beef by bending. If it cracks, remove and serve immediately. Or store in airtight container.

6. If still flexible, place back in dehydrator and continue dehydrating up to 4 hours, or until desired texture is achieved.

Fruit and Nut Apricot Pockets

Prep Time: 10 minutes

Servings: 4

INGREDIENTS

1 cup dried apricots

1/4 cup raw cashews

2 - 3 tablespoons dried cranberries

2 - 3 tablespoons dried blueberries

INSTRUCTIONS

1. Roughly chop cashews and add too small mixing bowl with cranberries and blueberries. Mix to combine.
2. Open apricots slightly to reveal pocket. Take pinch of mixed nuts and fruit and stuff apricots. Leave a little room to pinch apricot closed.
3. Transfer to serving dish and serve immediately. Or store in airtight container.

Sweet Treat Blondie Bars

Prep Time: 35 minutes

Servings: 6

INGREDIENTS

1 cup dried pitted dates

1 cup flaked or shredded coconut

3/4 cup golden flax seed

1/2 cup raw sunflower seeds (or raw pine nuts)

1/4 cup cacao butter (or coconut butter)

1/4 teaspoon Celtic sea salt

1 teaspoon vanilla

1/4cup cacao nibs (or raw chocolate chunks) (optional)

INSTRUCTIONS

1. Line baking dish with parchment paper. Allow cacao butter or coconut butter to soften.

2. Add flax to food processor or high-speed blender and process until finely ground, about 2 minutes. Add sunflower seeds and cacao butter. Process until fairly smooth, about 2 minutes.

3. Add dates, coconut, vanilla and salt. Process until mixture comes together, about 1 minute.

4. Transfer to medium mixing bowl and stir in cacao nibs or raw chocolate chunks (optional).

5. Transfer mixture to lined dish and press into bottom with hands or spatula. Place in freezer at least 25 minutes.

6. Remove from freezer. Slice and serve chilled. Or allow to warm slightly and serve.

Summer Sweet Bread

Prep Time: 10 minutes

Dehydrating Time: 6 - 8 hours

Servings: 8

INGREDIENTS

1 apple

1 lemon

1 orange

1 cup dried pitted dates

1/2 cup dried apricots

1/3 cup ground flax seed

1/2 cup raw pecans

1/2 cup raw walnuts

1 teaspoon ground cinnamon

1 teaspoon ground ginger

1/4 teaspoon Celtic sea salt

INSTRUCTIONS

1. Add pecans, walnuts and flax to food processor or high-speed blender. Process until finely ground, about 1 minute.

2. Peel and roughly chop apple around core. Zest *then* juice orange and lemon. Add to food processor or high-speed blender with dates, apricots, cinnamon, ginger and salt. Process until mixture is well ground and sticks together, about 2 minutes.

3. Line dehydrator tray with dehydrator or parchment sheet.

4. Form mixture into 2 loaves and place on lined dehydrator tray. Place in dehydrator and dehydrate at 115 degrees F for 2 hours. Reduce to 110 degrees F and continue to dehydrate for another 4 - 6 hours.

5. Remove from dehydrator and slice. Transfer to serving dish and serve immediately. Or store in airtight container.

Coconut Lemon Biscuits

Prep Time: 5 minutes

Dehydrating Time: 8 - 12 hours

Servings: 12

INGREDIENTS

1 cup cashews

1 cup flaked or shredded coconut

1 lemon

1 tablespoon raw honey

INSTRUCTIONS

1. Add cashews to food processor or high-speed blender and process until finely ground, about 1 minute.

2. Zest *then* juice lemon. Add to processor with coconut and honey. Process until mixture is well combined and sticks together, about 1 - 2 minutes.

3. Line dehydrator trays with dehydrator or parchment sheets.

4. Form mixture into 12 - 24 balls and place on dehydrator or parchment sheets. Press to flatten.

5. Place in dehydrator and dehydrate on 115 degrees F for about 8 - 12 hours, until desired crispiness is reached.

6. Remove from dehydrator and transfer to serving dish. Serve immediately. Or store in airtight container.

Spicy Sesame Crackers

Prep Time: 10 minutes

Dehydrating Time: 12 - 20 hours

Servings: 4

INGREDIENTS

2 cups ground flax seed

2/3 cup whole flax seed

1 1/3 cups raw sunflower seeds

1/2 cup raw black sesame seeds (or white sesame seeds)

1 orange

1 teaspoon ground cinnamon

1 teaspoon ground ginger

1 teaspoon ground black pepper (or ground white pepper)

1 teaspoon Celtic sea salt

2 2/3 cups water

INSTRUCTIONS

1. Place parchment paper or dehydrator sheets on dehydrator trays.

2. Zest *then* juice orange and add to large mixing bowl with water, seeds, salt and spices. Mix until well combined.

3. Spread batter on lined dehydrator trays. Place trays in dehydrator and set to 120 degrees F for 1 hour. Reduce temperature to 105 degrees F for 12 - 20.

4. After 4 hours, remove trays from dehydrator and use knife to score crackers in preferred shape and size. Place back in dehydrator and continue dehydrating.

5. Remove trays from dehydrator. Peel crackers from sheets and break apart along score lines. Place crackers directly on dehydrator tray and continue dehydrating another 6 - 12 hours, depending on desired crispness.

6. Remove crackers from dehydrator and serve immediately. Or store in an airtight container.

Cheesy Kale Crisps

Prep Time: 10 minutes

Cook Time: 12 - 24 hours

Servings: 8

INGREDIENTS

2 cups raw almonds

1 kale head (about 3 cups chopped)

1 cup raw coconut flour

1 cup golden flax seed

1 cup water

3/4 cup nutritional yeast

1/2 teaspoon ground black pepper

1 teaspoon smoked paprika

1 teaspoon Celtic sea salt

INSTRUCTIONS

1. Place parchment paper or dehydrator sheets on dehydrator trays.

2. Add flax to food processor or high-speed blender and process until finely ground, about 2 minutes. Transfer to small mixing bowl with water. Mix to combine and set aside.

3. Add almonds to food processor or high-speed blender and process until finely ground, about 2 minutes. Transfer to medium mixing bowl.

4. Wash and spin dry kale. Add to processor and pulse to finely chop, about 1 minute. Add to mixing bowl with nutritional yeast, salt and spices. Add soaked flax and mix until dough forms.

5. Transfer dough to lined dehydrator trays and press into 1/4 inch thick rectangle with hands or rolling pin. Score with knife or pizza cutter into desired shapes.

6. Place tray in dehydrator and dehydrate at 120 degrees F for 2 hours. Reduce temperature to 115 degrees F and continue to dehydrate for 8 - 12 hours.

7. After 6 hours, remove trays from dehydrator and flip crackers. Place back in dehydrator and continue dehydrating .

8. Remove crackers from dehydrator and serve immediately. Or store in airtight container.

Spicy Jalapeño Poppers

Prep Time: 20 minutes*

Dehydrating Time: 8 - 24 hours

Servings: 2

INGREDIENTS

6 fresh jalapeño peppers

Filling

1 cup raw sunflower seeds

1/2 cup water

1/4 cup nutritional yeast

1 lemon

1 teaspoon onion powder

1 teaspoon Celtic sea salt

Water

Breading

1/2 cup raw almonds

1/2 teaspoon Celtic sea salt

1/2 teaspoon ground white pepper (or ground black pepper)

1/2 teaspoon garlic powder (optional)

1/2 teaspoon onion powder (optional)

INSTRUCTIONS

1. *Soak sunflower seeds in enough water to cover for 2 hours. Drain and rinse.

2. Cut jalapeños in half lengthwise and remove stems, seeds and veins. Place peppers on dehydrator tray.

3. For *Filling*, juice lemon and add to food processor or high-speed blender with soaked sunflower seeds, water, nutritional yeast, salt, pepper and spices. Process until thick, smooth paste forms, about 2 minutes.

4. Fill piping bag with mixture and pipe into jalapeño halves. Or use teaspoon to scoop filling into jalapeño halves.

5. For *Breading*, add raw almonds to clean food processor orhigh-speed blender with salt and spices. Process until well ground but some texture remains, about 30 seconds.

6. Dip stuffed peppers filling-side down into bread and coat generously.

7. Place stuffed and coated peppers on dehydrator tray filling-side up. Place in dehydrator and dehydrate at 110 degrees F for 8 - 24 hours, depending on desired texture.

8. Remove peppers from dehydrator and serve immediately.

Savory Pepperdew Poppers

Prep Time: 15 minutes

Dehydrating Time: 4 - 8 hours

Servings: 2

INGREDIENTS

6 - 8 pepperdew peppers

Pine Nut Filling

1/4 cup raw tahini (or 6 tablespoons raw sesame seeds)

1/4 cup + 2 tablespoons raw pine nuts

1 tablespoon raw oil (coconut, walnut, almond, sesame, etc.)

1 tablespoon nutritional yeast

Juice of 1/2 lemon

1/2 teaspoon ground white pepper (or ground black pepper)

1/2 teaspoon Celtic sea salt

INSTRUCTIONS

1. Cut tops off of peppers and scoop out seeds. Set aside.
2. Add tahini or sesame seeds, 1/4 cup pine nuts, oil, nutritional yeast, lemon juice, salt and pepper to food processor or high-speed blender. Process until smooth and creamy, up to 5 minutes.
3. Scoop *Pine Nut Filling* into peppers and top with reserved pine nuts. Press pine nuts into stuffing to seal opening.
4. Place filled peppers in dehydrator and dehydrate at 110 degrees F for 4 - 8 hours, until dried but still moist.

5. Remove peppers from dehydrator and transfer to serving dish. Serve immediately. Or store in airtight container.

Fruity Granola Bars

Prep Time: 30 minutes

Servings: 8

INGREDIENTS

1 cup raw cashews (or 3/4 cup raw cashew butter)

2 tablespoons flax seed (or chia seed)

1/2 cup dried pitted dates

1/2 cup shredded or flaked coconut

1/3 cup raw pumpkin seeds

1/3 cup raw walnuts

1/3 cup raw almonds

1/4 cup dried cherries

1/4 cup dried blueberries

1/4cup dried raspberries

1/2 teaspoon ground ginger (optional)

1/2 teaspoon vanilla

1 teaspoon Celtic sea salt

INSTRUCTIONS

1. Line loaf pan with parchment paper.

2. Add flax or chia to food processor or high-speed blender and process until finely ground, about 1 - 2 minutes.

3. Add cashews (if using)and process until thick, smooth paste forms, up to 5 minutes.

4. Add dates and process until thick, fairly smooth mixture forms about 1 - 2 minutes. Transfer to medium mixing bowl.

5. Add coconut, pumpkin seeds, walnuts, almonds, vanilla, salt, dried fruit and ginger (optional). Add prepared cashew butter (if using). Stir to combine with large wooden spoon.

6. Transfer mixture to parchment lined pan and firmly press into bottom with hands or spatula. Place in refrigerator for 20 minutes.

7. Remove from refrigerator and cut into bars. Serve chilled. Or allow to warm to room temperature and serve.

Banana Berry Fruit Rolls

Prep Time: 5 minutes

Dehydrating Time: 6 hours

Servings: 6

INGREDIENTS

1 ripe banana

2 cups fresh strawberries (chopped)

2 tablespoons ground chia or flax seed (optional)

Water (optional)

INSTRUCTIONS

1. Remove stems from fresh strawberries and roughly chop. Peel and chop banana. Add to food processor or high-speed blender and process until smooth, about 1 minute.

2. Add ground chia or flax to processor and process with enough water to reach desired consistency. Mixture should be spreadable but not runny.

3. Line dehydrator tray with dehydrator or parchment sheet.

4. Spread mixture on sheet 1/4 inch thick in large rectangle with spatula. Place in dehydrator and dehydrate at 115 degrees F for 4 hours.

5. Remove from dehydrator and use offset spatula to gently peel leather from sheet and flip over. Place back in dehydrator directly on tray and continue to dehydrate for 2 hours.

6. Remove from dehydrator and cut into strips. Or roll up and cut into logs. Transfer to serving dish and serve immediately.

Crispy Carrot Chips

Prep Time: 5 minutes

Dehydrating Time: 18 - 24 hours

Servings: 4

INGREDIENTS

2 large carrots

1 tablespoon raw oil (coconut, walnut, almond, sesame, etc.) (optional)

1/2 teaspoon Celtic sea salt (optional)

INSTRUCTIONS

1. Carefully cut carrot into 1/16 - 1/8 inch thick slices with sharp knife, mandolin or food processor with slicing attachment.
2. Add sliced carrot to medium mixing bowl with oil and salt and toss to coat (optional).
3. Add single layer of sliced carrots to dehydrator tray and place in dehydrator. Dehydrate at 115 degrees F for 12 hours.
4. Remove dehydrator trays and turn over carrot slices. Place trays back in dehydrator and continue dehydrating for 6 - 12 hours, depending on desired crispiness.
5. Remove carrots from dehydrator and transfer to serving dish. Serve immediately. Or store in airtight container.

Acorn Squash Crisps

Prep Time: 5 minutes

Dehydrating Time: 18 - 24 hours

Servings: 4

INGREDIENTS

1 acorn squash

1 tablespoon raw oil (coconut, walnut, almond, sesame, etc.) (optional)

1/4 teaspoon smoked paprika

1/4 teaspoon ground white pepper (or ground black pepper)

1/4 teaspoon Italian seasoning blend (optional)

1/2 teaspoon Celtic sea salt

INSTRUCTIONS

1. Carefully cut acorn squash into 1/16 - 1/8 inch thick slices with sharp knife, mandolin or food processor with slicing attachment.

2. Add sliced squash to medium mixing bowl with oil, salt and spices. Toss to coat.

3. Add single layer of sliced squash to dehydrator tray and place in dehydrator. Dehydrate at 115 degrees F for 12 hours.

4. Remove dehydrator trays and turn over squash slices. Place trays back in dehydrator and continue dehydrating for 6 - 12 hours, depending on desired crispiness.

5. Remove squash from dehydrator and transfer to serving dish. Serve immediately. Or store in airtight container.

Confetti Beet Chips

Prep Time: 15 minutes

Dehydrating Time: 18 - 24 hours

Servings: 4

INGREDIENTS

2 red beets

2 golden beets (or 2 red beets)

1/4 cup water

1/4 cup raw apple cider vinegar

1 tablespoon raw oil (coconut, walnut, almond, sesame, etc.)

1 teaspoon Celtic seat salt

1/2 teaspoon ground black pepper

INSTRUCTIONS

1. Wash and scrub beets. Carefully cut into 1/16 - 1/8 inch thick slices with sharp knife, mandolin or food processor with slicing attachment.

2. Add sliced beets to medium mixing bowl with water, vinegar and oil. Toss to coat. Set aside 10 minutes.

3. Drain beets, then sprinkle on salt and pepper. Toss to coat.

4. Add single layer of beets to dehydrator tray and place in dehydrator. Dehydrate at 115 degrees F for 12 hours.

5. Remove dehydrator trays and turn over beet slices. Place trays back in dehydrator and continue dehydrating for 12 hours, depending on desired crispiness.

6. Remove beets from dehydrator and transfer to serving dish. Serve immediately. Or store in airtight container.

Mango Snacks

Prep Time: 10 minutes

Dehydrating Time: 24 hours

Servings: 4

INGREDIENTS

2 ripe mangos

INSTRUCTIONS

1. Cut mango around pit, and cut into 1/4 inch thick slices. Then remove peel. Or slice then peel.
2. Add single layer of sliced mango to dehydrator trays. Place in dehydrator and dehydrate at 115 degrees F for 24 hours, or until dried but not crisp.
3. Remove mango from dehydrator and transfer to serving dish. Serve immediately. Or store in airtight container.

Pineapple Chews

Prep Time: 10 minutes

Dehydrating Time: 12 - 16 hours

Servings: 4

INGREDIENTS

1 ripe pineapple

INSTRUCTIONS

1. Peel pineapple and cut around core into 1/4 - 1/3 inch thick slices.
2. Add single layer of sliced pineapple to dehydrator trays. Place in dehydrator and dehydrate at 115 degrees F for 12 - 16 hours, or until dried but not crisp.
3. Remove pineapple from dehydrator and transfer to serving dish. Serve immediately. Or store in airtight container.

Banana Crisps

Prep Time: 5 minutes

Dehydrating Time: 12 - 16 hours

Servings: 4

INGREDIENTS

4 ripe or overripe bananas

INSTRUCTIONS

1. Peel bananas and cut into 1/4 - 1/3 inch thick slices lengthwise or crosswise.
2. Line dehydrator trays with dehydrator or parchment sheet. Add single layer of sliced banana to lined dehydrator trays .
3. Place bananas in dehydrator and dehydrate on 115 degrees F for 12 - 16 hours, depending on desired crispiness.
4. Remove bananas from dehydrator and transfer to serving dish. Serve immediately. Or store in airtight container.

Sweet Apple Chips

Prep Time: 5 minutes

Dehydrating Time: 10 - 14 hours

Servings: 4

INGREDIENTS

4 sweet apples

1 teaspoon ground cinnamon (optional)

INSTRUCTIONS

1. Carefully cut apple around core into 1/16 - 1/8 inch thick slices with sharp knife, mandolin or food processor with slicing attachment.
2. Add single layer of sliced apple to dehydrator tray . Sprinkle with cinnamon (optional). Place in dehydrator and dehydrate at 105 degrees F for 10 - 14 hours, depending on desired crispiness.
3. Remove apples from dehydrator and transfer to serving dish. Serve immediately. Or store in airtight container.

Spicy Kale Crisps

Prep Time: 10 minutes

Dehydrating Time: 4 - 6 hours

Servings: 4

INGREDIENTS

2 kale heads (or 1.5 - 2 lbs kale leaves)

3 tablespoons raw oil (coconut, walnut, almond, sesame, etc.)

1 tablespoon coconut aminos (or tamari, apple cider vinegar or lemon juice)

1/2 teaspoon smoked paprika

1 teaspoon cayenne pepper

1 teaspoon ground black pepper

1 teaspoon Celtic sea salt

INSTRUCTIONS

1. Wash and spin dry kale. Remove tough spine and chop or tear into pieces.
2. Add kale pieces to large mixing bowl with oil, vinegar salt and spices. Toss to coat.
3. Add single layer of coated kale to dehydrator tray and place in dehydrator. Dehydrate at 115 degrees F for 4 - 6 hours, depending on desired crispiness.
4. Remove kale from dehydrator and transfer to serving dish. Serve immediately. Or store in airtight container.

Savory Sweet Potato Chips

Prep Time: 5 minutes

Dehydrating Time: 24 hours

Servings: 4

INGREDIENTS

1 large sweet potato

2 tablespoons raw oil (coconut, walnut, almond, sesame, etc.)

1 teaspoon Celtic sea salt

1/2 teaspoon ground black pepper (optional)

INSTRUCTIONS

1. Carefully cut sweet potato into 1/16 - 1/8 inch thick slices with sharp knife, mandolin or food processor with slicing attachment.
2. Add sliced sweet potato to medium mixing bowl with oil, salt and pepper. Toss to coat.
3. Add single layer of coated sweet potatoes to dehydrator tray and place in dehydrator. Dehydrate at 115 degrees F for 12 hours.
4. Remove dehydrator trays and turn over sweet potato slices. Place trays back in dehydrator and continue dehydrating for about 12 hours, depending on desired crispiness.
5. Remove sweet potatoes from dehydrator and transfer to serving dish. Serve immediately. Or store in airtight container.

Cheesy Popcorn

Prep Time: 5 minutes

Dehydrating Time: 12 - 24 hours

Servings: 2

INGREDIENTS

2 cups cauliflower florets (roughly chopped)

1 teaspoon raw oil (coconut, walnuts, almond, sesame, etc.)

1 teaspoon coconut aminos (or tamari, apple cider vinegar or lemon juice)

3 tablespoons nutritional yeast

1 teaspoon Celtic sea salt

INSTRUCTIONS

1. Cut larger cauliflower florets into smaller pieces. Add to medium mixing bowl or container with well-fitting lid.
2. Evenly sprinkle on oil, coconut aminos, nutritional yeast and salt.
3. Secure lid on bowl or container and shake well until cauliflower is evenly coated.
4. Line dehydrator trays with dehydrator or parchment sheets.
5. Add single layer of coated cauliflower to lined dehydrator trays and place in dehydrator. Dehydrate at 115 degrees F for 12 - 24 hours, until desired crispiness is reached. Turn cauliflower over half way through dehydrating.
6. Remove from dehydrator and transfer to serving dish. Serve immediately.

Kids Recipes

Easy Chocolate Milk

Prep Time: 5 minutes*

Servings: 2

INGREDIENTS

1 cup raw almonds

1/4 cup raw honey (dried pitted dates)

2 - 3 tablespoons raw cocoa powder

1/2 teaspoon vanilla

Water

INSTRUCTIONS

1. *Soak almonds in enough water to cover at least 6 hours, or overnight in refrigerator. Drain and rinse. Soak dates in enough water to cover at least 6 hours, or overnight in refrigerator. Drain.

2. Add almonds and dates (if using) to high-speed blender with 3 cups water. Process until well blended and almost smooth, about 1 - 2 minutes.

3. Strain mixture through nut milk bag, cheesecloth or strainer back into blender. Reserve pulp and set aside to dry and dehydrate, then use as almond flour.

4. Add cocoa, vanilla and honey (if using) to blender and process until emulsified, about 1 - 2 minutes.

5. Pour into glasses and serve immediately. Or refrigerate 20 minutes and serve chilled. Process or stir to reincorporate if cocoa separates from milk.

Stuffed Apple Snack

Prep Time: 10 minutes

Servings: 2

INGREDIENTS

2 apples

Almond Butter

1 cup raw almonds

1 teaspoon raw oil (almond, coconut, walnut, etc.) (optional)

1 teaspoon raw honey

1/4 teaspoon Celtic sea salt

Pinch ground cinnamon

INSTRUCTIONS

1. Add almonds to food processor or high-speed blender. Process until smooth, up to 10 minutes. Scrape down sides as needed. Add oil to reach desired consistency (optional).

2. Add honey, salt and cinnamon and process to incorporate, about 30 seconds.

3. Remove core, seeds and stems from apples. Leave apples hollow in center.

4. Scoop *Almond Butter* into hollowed apples with small spoon or knife. Fill hollows completely and transfer stuffed apples to serving dish.

5. Serve immediately. Or refrigerate 20 minutes and serve chilled.

Cashew Cream and Carrots

Prep Time: 5 minutes*

Servings: 2

INGREDIENTS

2 large carrots

Cashew Cream

1 cup raw cashews

4 dried pitted dates

1/2 teaspoon ground cinnamon

1/4 teaspoon Celtic sea salt

Pinch ground ginger

Water (or raw nut milk)

INSTRUCTIONS

1. *Soak cashews in enough water to cover at least 6 hours, or overnight in refrigerator. Drain and rinse. Soak dates in enough water to cover at least 6 hours, or overnight in refrigerator. Drain.

2. Add cashews, dates, cinnamon, salt and ginger to food processor or high-speed blender. Process until smooth, about 2 minutes. Add enough water or raw nut milk to reach desired consistency. Transfer to serving dish.

3. Cut carrots into sticks and transfer to serving dish.

4. Serve carrots with *Cashew Cream* immediately. Or refrigerate 20 minutes and serve chilled.

Chocolate Spread on Celery

Prep Time: 10 minutes*

Servings: 2

INGREDIENTS

2 - 3 medium celery stalks

Hazelnut Spread

1 cup raw hazelnuts

1/4 cup raw cocoa powder

1/4 cup raw honey (or dried pitted dates)

1/2 teaspoon vanilla

Pinch Celtic sea salt

Raw nut milk (optional)

Water

INSTRUCTIONS

1. *Soak hazelnuts in enough water to cover overnight in refrigerator. Drain and rinse. Soak dates in enough water to cover overnight in refrigerator, if using. Drain.

2. Add soaked hazelnuts to food processor or high-speed blender and process until smooth, up to 10 minutes. Scrape down sides as needed.

3. Add honey or soaked dates, cocoa powder, vanilla and salt to processor. Process until smooth, about 1 minute. Add nut milk to reach desired consistency (optional).

7. Cut celery stalks into 3 in pieces. Scoop *Hazelnut Spread* into wells of celery with small spoon or knife. Fill wells completely and smooth with knife or back of spoon. Transfer filled celery to serving dish.

8. Serve immediately. Or refrigerate 20 minutes and serve chilled.

Cashew Apple Stack

Prep Time: 5 minutes

Servings: 2

INGREDIENTS

1 apple

Cashew Butter

1 cup raw cashews

2 dried pitted dates

1 teaspoon raw oil (coconut, walnut, almond, sesame, etc.) (optional)

1/4 teaspoon ground cinnamon

Pinch Celtic sea salt

INSTRUCTIONS

1. For *Cashew Butter*, add cashews, dates, cinnamon, salt and oil (optional) to food processor or high-speed blender. Process until smooth, up to 5 minutes. Let mixture rest between periods of processing to reach desired consistency, if necessary.

2. Thinly slice apple around core and stem with knife or mandolin. Place slices of apple on serving dish and top with dollop of *Cashew Butter*. Place another apple slice on *Cashew Butter*, and repeat until apple slices and *Cashew Butter* are used.

3. Serve immediately. Or refrigerate for 20 minutes and serve chilled.

Simple Banana Pudding

Prep Time: 10 minutes

Servings: 2

INGREDIENTS

Banana Pudding

1 large overripe banana (or 2 small overripe bananas)

1/2 cup raw cashews

1/4 cup dried pitted dates

1 lemon

2 tablespoons raw coconut butter (or cacao butter or coconut oil)

1/2 teaspoon vanilla

Pinch Celtic sea salt

Vanilla Crumbles

1/4 cup raw cashews

2 tablespoons flaked or shredded coconut

2 dried pitted dates

Pinch vanilla

Pinch Celtic sea salt

INSTRUCTIONS

1. For *Banana Pudding*, juice lemon and add to food processor or high-speed blender with dates. Process until well ground, about 1 minute.
2. Add cashews and process until smooth, up to 5 minutes.

3. Peel banana and add to processor with coconut butter, vanilla and salt. Process until creamy and smooth, about 1 - 2 minutes.
4. Transfer mixture to serving dish.
5. For *Vanilla Crumbles*, add cashews, coconut, dates, vanilla and salt to clean food processor or high-speed blender. Pulse until crumbly mixture forms.
6. Top *Banana Pudding* with *Vanilla Crumbles* and serve immediately. Or refrigerate for 20 minutes and serve chilled.

True Chocolate Pudding

Prep Time: 10 minutes*

Servings: 2

INGREDIENTS

1 1/2 cups raw cashews

1/2 cup flaked or shredded coconut

1/2 cup dried pitted dates

1/4 cup raw cacao powder

1 teaspoon vanilla

Water

INSTRUCTIONS

1. *Soak cashews and dates in enough water to cover overnight in refrigerator. Drain. Separately soak coconut in 3/4 cup water overnight in refrigerator.

2. Add soaked coconut and soaking liquid to high-speed blender. Process until fairly smooth, about 1 - 2 minutes.

3. Strain mixture through nut milk bag, cheesecloth or strainer back into blender or into food processor. Dry coconut pulp, process until finely ground, and use as coconut flour.

4. Add soaked cashews and dates, cocoa and vanilla to coconut milk. Process until smooth and creamy, up to 5 minutes.

5. Transfer to serving dish and serve immediately. Or refrigerate or freeze 20 minutes, then serve chilled.

Afterschool Applesauce

Prep Time: 5 minutes

Servings: 2

INGREDIENTS

2 large apples

1 tablespoon lemon juice (or apple cider vinegar)

1/2 teaspoon vanilla (optional)

1/2 teaspoon cinnamon (optional)

INSTRUCTIONS

1. Peel apples, if preferred. Remove core, seeds and stem, then roughly chop. Add to food processor or high-speed blender with lemon juice, vanilla and cinnamon (optional). Process until smooth, about 1 - 2 minutes. Scrape down as necessary.
2. Transfer to serving dish and serve immediately. Or refrigerate for 20 minutes and serve chilled.

Almond Butter and Jelly Bars

Prep Time: 30 minutes

Servings: 6

INGREDIENTS

Almond Butter Bars

1 1/2 cups raw almonds (or 1 cup raw almond butter)

1/2 cup dried pitted dates

1/3 cup shredded or flaked coconut

2 tablespoons chia seeds (or flax seeds)

2 tablespoon raw oil (almond, walnut, coconut, sesame, etc.)

1 teaspoon vanilla

1 teaspoon Celtic sea salt

Strawberry Jelly

1 cup fresh strawberries

1/2 cup dried strawberries

1 orange

1/2 teaspoon vanilla

INSTRUCTIONS

1. Line baking dish with parchment paper.
2. For *Strawberry Jelly*, juice orange and add to small bowl with dried strawberries. Set aside 5 - 10 minutes
3. For *Almond Butter Bar*, add chia or flax to food processor or high-speed blender. Process until well ground, about 2 minutes.

4. Add almonds and oil to processor and process until smooth, up to 5 minutes. Or add prepared almond butter and oil to processor and process about 30 seconds.

5. Add dates, vanilla and salt and process until mixture sticks together, about 2 minutes. Stir in coconut.

6. Transfer mixture to lined baking dish and press firmly into bottom with hands or spatula. Place in refrigerator and chill for 10 minutes.

7. Remove stems from fresh strawberries and roughly chop. Add to clean food processor or high-speed blender with vanilla, soaked fruit and juice. Process until mostly smooth, about 1 minute..

8. Remove *Almond Butter Bars* from refrigerator and spread on *Strawberry Jelly*. Slice and serve immediately.

Pecan Brownies

Prep Time: 10 minutes*

Servings: 6

INGREDIENTS

1 cup raw pecans

1 cup dried pitted dates

2 tablespoons raw coconut butter (or cacao butter)

1/4 cup raw cocoa powder

1/4 cup shredded or flaked coconut

1/4 teaspoon Celtic sea salt

INSTRUCTIONS

1. Line square baking dish with parchment paper. Allow coconut or cacao butter to soften.

2. Add pecans to food processor or high-speed blender and process until finely ground, about 1 minute.

3. Add dates and coconut or cacao butter and process until mixture sticks together, about 1 - 2 minutes.

4. Add cocoa, coconut and salt. Process until well ground but not completely smooth.

5. *Transfer mixture to parchment lined baking dish and firmly press into bottom with hands or spatula. Refrigerate until set, about 2 hours.

6. Remove from refrigerator. Slice and serve chilled. Or allow to warm to room temperature and serve.

Chocolate Chip Cookie Dough Bites

Prep Time: 35 minutes

Servings: 6

INGREDIENTS

1 1/4 cups fine almond flour

3 teaspoons coconut flour

1/3 cup dried pitted dates

1/4 cup raw coconut butter (or cacao butter)

1 teaspoon vanilla

1/8 teaspoon Celtic sea salt

1/2 cup raw chocolate chips (or chopped raw chocolate bark or cacao nibs)

INSTRUCTIONS

1. Allow coconut or cacao butter to soften at room temperature. Line sheet pan with parchment paper.
2. Add softened butter and dates to food processor or high speed blender. Process until fairly smooth, about 2 minutes.
3. Add half of almond and coconut flours, and process for about 1 minute. Add remaining flour, vanilla and salt. Process until mixture comes together. Stir in chocolate or cacao nibs.
4. Use tablespoon or mini ice cream scoop to form dough into balls. Set on lined sheet pan and place in refrigerator 30 minutes.
5. Remove from refrigerator and serve chilled. Or allow to warm slightly and serve room temperature.

Super Fruit Granola Bars

Prep Time: 30 minutes

Servings: 8

INGREDIENTS

1 cup raw cashews (or 3/4 cup raw cashew butter)

2 tablespoons flax seed (or chia seed)

1/2 cup dried pitted dates

1/2 cup shredded or flaked coconut

1/3 cup raw pumpkin seeds

1/3 cup raw walnuts

1/3 cup raw almonds

1/4 cup raw chocolate chips (or cacao nibs)

1/4 cup dried goji or noni berries (optional)

1/2 teaspoon ground cinnamon

1/2 teaspoon vanilla

1 teaspoon Celtic sea salt

INSTRUCTIONS

1. Line loaf pan with parchment paper.
2. Add flax or chia to food processor or high-speed blender and process until finely ground, about 1 - 2 minutes.
3. Add cashews (if using)and process until thick, smooth paste forms, up to 5 minutes.
4. Add dates and process until thick, fairly smooth mixture forms about 1 - 2 minutes. Transfer to medium mixing bowl.

5. Add coconut, pumpkin seeds, walnuts, almonds, cinnamon, vanilla, salt, chocolate chips or cacao nibs, and goji or noni berries (optional). Add prepared cashew butter (if using). Stir to combine with large wooden spoon.

6. Transfer mixture to parchment lined pan and firmly press into bottom with hands or spatula. Place in refrigerator for 20 minutes.

7. Remove from refrigerator and cut into bars. Serve chilled. Or allow to warm to room temperature and serve.

Awesome Chocolate Fudge

Prep Time: 10 minutes*

Servings: 6

INGREDIENTS

1 cup raw cashew butter (or 1 1/2 raw cashews)

1/3 cup raw cacao butter (or coconut butter or oil)

1/4 cup cocoa powder

1/4 cup raw honey

1 teaspoon vanilla

1/2 teaspoon Celtic sea salt

INSTRUCTIONS

1. Line loaf pan with parchment paper.
2. Add cashews and cacao butter to food processor or high-speed blender and process until smooth, up to 5 minutes.
3. Or add prepared cashew butter, cacao butter, cocoa powder, honey, vanilla and salt to food processor, high-speed blender or small mixing bowl. Process or mix until combined.
4. Transfer to parchment lined dish and smooth with spatula. Place in freezer at least 1 hour.
5. Remove from freezer. Slice and serve immediately. Or allow to warm slightly and serve.

Strawberry Fruit Rolls

Prep Time: 15 minutes

Dehydrating Time: 6 hours

Servings: 6

INGREDIENTS

1 cup dried strawberries

2 cups fresh strawberries

2 tablespoons ground chia or flax seed (optional)

Water (optional)

INSTRUCTIONS

1. Remove stems from fresh strawberries and roughly chop. Add to food processor or high-speed blender and process until smooth, about 30 seconds.

2. Add dried strawberries and process until smooth, about 1 minute. Set aside 10 minutes.

3. Add ground chia or flax to processor and process with enough water to reach desired consistency. Mixture should be spreadable but not runny.

4. Line dehydrator tray with dehydrator or parchment sheet.

5. Spread mixture on sheet 1/4 inch thick in large rectangle with spatula. Place in dehydrator and dehydrate on 115 degrees F for 4 hours.

6. Remove from dehydrator and use offset spatula to gently peel leather from sheet and flip over. Place back in dehydrator and continue to dehydrate for 2 hours.
7. Remove from dehydrator and cut into strips. Or roll up and cut into logs. Transfer to serving dish and serve immediately.

Chocolate Banana Pops

Prep Time: 30 minutes

Servings: 4

INGREDIENTS

1 large banana

Chocolate Coating

1/2 cup coconut oil (liquid)

1/4 cup raw honey (or coconut sap)

1/4 cup raw cocoa powder

Toothpicks, popsicle or lollipop sticks

INSTRUCTIONS

1. Linc small baking dish or plate with parchment paper. Plate in freeze at least 5 minutes.
2. Add coconut oil, cocoa and honey to food processor, high-speed blender or small mixing bowl. Process or whisk until emulsified, about 15 - 60 seconds.
3. Peel banana and cut into 1 1/2 inch slices. Insert toothpicks, popsicle or lollipop sticks into banana pieces.
4. Remove parchment lines dish from freezer.
5. Dip banana pieces into cocoa mixture. Coat well and transfer to lined dish.
6. Place in freeze at least 20 minutes, until coating is hard and banana is frozen.

7. For thicker *Chocolate Coating*, dip frozen *Banana Pops* back into *Chocolate Coating* and freeze another 5 minutes.

8. Remove from freezer and transfer to serving dish. Serve immediately.

Orange Cream Popsicles

Prep Time: 10 minutes*

Servings: 12

INGREDIENTS

2 cups orange or tangerine juice (about 9 oranges or 15 tangerines)

1/2 cup shredded or flaked coconut (or 1 mature coconut)

Water

Ice pop maker, toothpicks or popsicle sticks

INSTRUCTIONS

1. *Freeze ice pop maker or ice cube tray for at least 30 minutes.
2. *Soak flaked coconut in 2/3 - 3/4 cups water at least 6 hours, or overnight in refrigerator.
3. Add soaked coconut and soaking liquid to food processor or high-speed blender.
4. Or remove flesh from fresh coconut and add to high-speed blender with 2/3 - 3/4 cups water. Process until well blended and fairly smooth, about 1 - 2 minutes.
5. Strain mixture through nut milk bag, cheesecloth or strainer back into blender. Reserve pulp and set aside to dry and dehydrate, then use as coconut flour.
6. Juice oranges and add to blender. Process until well combined, about 30 seconds.
7. Remove ice pop maker or ice cube tray from freezer. Pour mixture into wells and fill 3/4 full. Place in freezer about 20 minutes.

8. Place ice pop maker sticks, toothpicks or popsicle sticks into well. Return to freezer about 20 minutes.

9. Remove ice pops from freezer and serve immediately.

Sweet Coconut Ice Cream

Prep Time: 30 minutes*

Servings: 4

INGREDIENTS

2 1/2 cups shredded or flaked coconut (or 3 mature coconuts + 1/2 cups shredded or flaked coconut)

3/4 cup dried pitted dates (or raw honey)

1 1/2 teaspoons vanilla

Water

INSTRUCTIONS

1. *Freeze ice cream maker canister for at least 12 hours.
2. *Soak 2 cups coconut in 4 cups water at least 6 hours, or overnight in refrigerator. Soak dates in enough water to cover at least 6 hours, or overnight in refrigerator (if using). Drain.
3. Add soaked coconut, soaking liquid and dates (if using) to food processor or high-speed blender.
4. Or remove flesh from fresh coconuts and add to high-speed blender with 4 cups water and dates (if using). Process until well blended and fairly smooth, about 1 - 2 minutes.
5. Strain mixture through nut milk bag, cheesecloth or strainer back into blender. Reserve pulp and set aside to dry and dehydrate, then use as coconut flour.
6. Add 1/2 cup shredded or flaked coconut, vanilla and honey (if using) to coconut milk. Process to combine, about 10 seconds.

7. Assemble ice cream maker and turn on. Slowly pour mixture into running ice cream maker. Let machine run for about 20 minutes, until ice cream is set.

8. Transfer to serving dish and serve immediately.

Lemonade Slush

Prep Time: 5 minutes

Servings: 2

INGREDIENTS

1 cup fresh lemon juice (about 6 lemons)

1/4 - 1/3 cup raw honey

1 cup ice (preferably crushed)

1/4 teaspoon vanilla (optional)

INSTRUCTIONS

1. Juice lemons and add to food processor or high-speed blender with ice, honey and vanilla (optional). Process until well blended and smooth, about 1 - 2 minutes.
2. Transfer to serving dish and serve immediately.

Cherry Crush

Prep Time: 5 minutes

Servings: 2

INGREDIENTS

1 cup pitted cherries (fresh or frozen)

2 oranges

1/2 cup ice (preferably crushed)

1/4 teaspoon vanilla (optional)

Water (optional)

INSTRUCTIONS

1. Pit cherries, if fresh. Juice oranges.
2. Add orange juice, cherries, ice and vanilla (optional) to high-speed blender. Process until smooth, about 1 minute. Add enough water to reach desired consistency (optional).
3. Pour into glasses and serve immediately.

Sweet Potato Sticks

Prep Time: 25 minutes

Dehydrating Time: 7 - 10 hours

Servings: 2

INGREDIENTS

1 large sweet potato

1/2 tablespoon raw oil (coconut, walnut, almond, sesame, etc.)

1/2 teaspoon ground black pepper

1/2 teaspoon Celtic sea salt

Raw Ketchup

1 plum tomato

1/4 cup sundried tomatoes

2 dried pitted dates (or 1 tablespoon raw honey)

2 teaspoons raw apple cider vinegar

1/4 teaspoon onion powder

1/4 teaspoon garlic powder

1/4 teaspoon Celtic sea salt

INSTRUCTIONS

1. Cut sweet potato into strips of desired thickness. Add to medium mixing bowl or container with well-fitting lid.

2. Evenly sprinkle on oil, salt and pepper. Secure lid on bowl or container and shake well until sweet potato is evenly coated. Set aside 20 minutes.

3. Line dehydrator trays with dehydrator or parchment sheets.

4. Add single layer of coated sweet potatoes to lined dehydrator sheet and place in dehydrator. Dehydrate on 125 degrees F for 2 hours. Reduce temperature to 110 degrees F and continue dehydrating for 5 - 8 hours, depending on desired crispiness.

5. For *Raw Ketchup*, soak sundried tomatoes and dates (if using) in enough water to cover for at least 1 hour. Drain and reserve 2 teaspoons soaking liquid.

6. Add soaked sundried tomatoes and dates, reserved liquid, plum tomato, vinegar, salt, spices and honey (if using) to food processor or high-speed blender. Process until smooth, about 1 - 2 minutes. Transfer to serving dish.

7. Remove sweet potatoes from dehydrator and transfer to serving dish. Serve immediately with *Raw Ketchup*.

Crispy Onion Rings

Prep Time: 15 minutes*

Dehydrating Time: 16 - 24 hours

Servings: 4

INGREDIENTS

Almond Milk/Coating

1/2 cup raw almonds

Water

Onions Rings

2 cups *Almond Milk*

1/3 cup *Almond Coating*

1 medium onion (sweet or white)

1/4 cup ground flax seed (or 1/3 cup whole flax seeds)

1 teaspoon smoked paprika

1/4 teaspoon ground white pepper (or pinch ground black pepper)

1/4 teaspoon Celtic sea salt

INSTRUCTIONS

1. *For *Almond Milk/Coating*, soak almonds in enough water to cover at least 6 hours, or overnight in refrigerator. Drain and pop off skins, if preferred.

2. Add soaked almonds to high-speed blender with 2 cups water. Process until well blended and almost smooth, about 1- 2 minutes.

3. Strain mixture through nut milk bag, cheesecloth or strainer into medium lidded container. Reserve almond pulp.

4. For *Almond Coating* Line dehydrator tray with dehydrator or parchment sheets. Spread almond pulp on lined dehydrator tray and dehydrate into on 110 degrees F for 6 - 12 hours, until completely dry.

5. Peel and slice onion. Add to *Almond Milk* and gently mix to coat. Let onions soak while *Almond Coating* dehydrates.

6. Remove *Almond Coating* from dehydrator and set aside. Line dehydrator trays with dehydrator or parchment sheets.

7. Add flax to food processor or high-speed blender with 1/3 cup *Almond Coating*, salt and spices. Process until finely ground. Split into 2 batches and transfer to shallow dishes.

8. Drain onions, reserving *Almond Milk*. Dip onions into *Almond Milk*, then *Almond Coating* mixture. For heavier coating, repeat.

9. Place coated onions in single layer on line dehydrator trays. Dehydrate on 110 degrees F for 6 - 8 hours, until *Almond Coating* is dry but onions are slightly moist.

10. Transfer to serving dish and serve immediately with your favorite sauce.

Cauliflower Popcorn

Prep Time: 5 minutes

Dehydrating Time: 12 - 24 hours

Servings: 2

INGREDIENTS

2 cups cauliflower florets (roughly chopped)

1 teaspoon raw oil (coconut, walnuts, almond, sesame, etc.)

1 tablespoon nutritional yeast

Celtic sea salt, to taste

Pinch cayenne pepper (optional)

INSTRUCTIONS

1. Cut larger cauliflower florets into smaller pieces. Add to medium mixing bowl or container with well-fitting lid.
2. Evenly sprinkle on oil, nutritional yeast, salt and cayenne pepper (optional).
3. Secure lid on bowl or container and shake well until cauliflower is evenly coated.
4. Line dehydrator trays with dehydrator or parchment sheets.
5. Add single layer of coated cauliflower to lined dehydrator sheet and place in dehydrator. Dehydrate on 115 degrees F for 12 - 24 hours, until desired crispiness is reached. Turn cauliflower over half way through ehydrating.
6. Remove from dehydrator and transfer to serving dish. Serve immediately.

Zucchini Lasagna Roll Ups

Prep Time: 15 minutes*

Servings: 4

INGREDIENTS

1 small zucchini

Water

Tomato Sauce

1/2 cup sundried tomatoes

2 plum tomato

1 dried pitted date

1 small garlic clove

1 teaspoon lemon juice

1/4 teaspoon dried basil

1/4 teaspoon dried oregano

Pinch ground black pepper

Cashew Cheese

1/3 cup raw cashews

1 small garlic clove

1/2 teaspoon lemon juice

1/4 Celtic sea salt

Walnut Sausage

1 cups raw walnuts

1 tablespoon coconut aminos (or tamari or raw apple cider vinegar)

1/2 teaspoon dried sage

1/2 teaspoon dried thyme

1/2 teaspoon fresh rosemary (optional)

1/4 teaspoon Celtics sea salt

INSTRUCTIONS

1. Separately soak cashews, walnuts, and sundried tomatoes and date in enough water to cover at least 6 hours, or overnight in refrigerator. Drain sundried tomatoes and date. Drain and rinse nuts.

2. For *Tomato Sauce*, peel garlic and add to food processor or high-speed blender with soaked tomatoes and date, fresh tomato, spices and lemon juice. Process until finely ground and fairly smooth, about 1 - 2 minutes. Add enough water to reach desired consistency, if necessary. Set aside.

3. For *Cashew Cheese*, peel garlic and add to clean food processor or high-speed blender with soaked cashews, salt and lemon juice. Process until smooth, about 2 minutes. Add enough water to reach desired consistency, if necessary. Set aside.

4. For *Walnut Sausage*, add soaked walnuts, coconut aminos, salt and spices to clean food processor or high-speed blender. Process until coarsely ground, about 1 minute. Set aside.

5. Carefully slice zucchini lengthwise into 1/8 - 1/4 inch long strips with knife or mandolin. Place layer of zucchini on serving dish. Layer *Tomato Sauce, Cashew Cheese* and *Walnut Sausage* on first 2 inches of zucchini strip.

6. Roll up zucchini of filling into tight log. Transfer to serving dish. Repeat with remaining ingredients.

7. Serve immediately. Or place in refrigerator for 20 minutes and serve chilled.

Squash Blossom Poppers

Prep Time: 10 minutes*

Dehydrating Time: 3 - 6 hours

Servings: 8

INGREDIENTS

16 squash blossoms

1/2 cup raw walnuts

1 avocado

1/2 small white onion

1/2 lemon

2 tablespoons nutritional yeast

1/2 teaspoon paprika

1/2 teaspoon ground white pepper (or ground black pepper)

1/2 teaspoon Celtic sea salt

1 tablespoon raw oil (walnuts, almond, coconut sesame, etc.)

2 tablespoons ground flax seeds

Water

INSTRUCTIONS

1. *Gently rinse blossoms and pat dry. Let air dry for 30 minutes.
2. Cut avocado in half and remove pit. Scoop flesh into food processor or high-speed blender with walnuts, squeeze of lemon, salt, pepper and spices. Process until smooth, about 2 minutes. Add enough water to reach desired consistency.
3. Peel onion and mince. Add to small mixing bowl with avocado mixture. Mix to combine. Spoon mixture into squash blossoms.

4. Line dehydrator tray with dehydrator or parchment sheet.

5. Finely grind flax seeds. Brush stuffed blossoms with oil and sprinkle with ground flax.

6. Transfer to lined dehydrator tray and place in dehydrator. Dehydrate on 115 degrees F for 3 - 6 hours, until flax coating is dried and blossoms appear "fried."

7. Remove from dehydrator and transfer to serving dish. Serve immediately.

Meatballs and Tomato Sauce

Prep Time: 10 minutes*

Dehydrating Time: 2 - 4 hours

Servings: 4

INGREDIENTS

Meatballs

1 cup raw walnuts

1 cup raw sunflower seeds

1 cup raw almonds

1 small celery stalk

1 large red bell pepper

1/4 small onion

2 garlic cloves

Medium bunch fresh parsley

1 spring fresh rosemary

1 teaspoon ground cumin

1 teaspoon Celtic sea salt

Pinch red pepper flakes (or cayenne pepper)

Water

Tomato Sauce

3 plum tomatoes

5 sundried tomatoes

2 tablespoons raw cashews (or 1 tablespoon raw cashew butter)

1 garlic clove

1/2 teaspoon dried basil

1/2 teaspoon dried oregano

Pinch ground black pepper

Pinch Celtic sea salt

INSTRUCTIONS

1. *For *Meatballs*, soak walnuts, almonds and sunflower seeds in enough water to cover for 2 hours. Drain.
2. Line dehydrator tray with dehydrator or parchment sheet.
3. Peel garlic and onion. Remove stem, seeds and veins from bell pepper. Chop garlic, onion, pepper, celery. Add to food processor or high-speed blender with soaked nuts, salt and spices. Process until well ground, about 2 minutes. Add enough water to reach desired consistency.
4. Form mixture into rounds with mini ice cram scoop or hands. Place on lined dehydrator tray. Dehydrate on 110 degrees F for 2 - 4 hour, until set and firm.
5. For *Tomato Sauce*, peel garlic and add to food processor or high-speed blender with tomatoes, sundried tomatoes, cashews or cashew butter, salt, pepper and spices. Process until smooth, about 1 - 2 minutes.
6. Remove *Meatballs* from dehydrator and transfer to serving dish. Top with *Tomato Sauce* and serve immediately.

Snacks Recipes

Crisp Sesame Crackers

Prep Time: 10 minutes

Dehydrating Time: 12 - 20 hours

Servings: 4

INGREDIENTS

2 cups ground flax seed

2/3 cup whole flax seed

1 1/3 cups raw sunflower seeds

1/2 cup raw black sesame seeds (or white sesame seeds)

Small bunch fresh parsley

1/4 teaspoon dried basil

1/4 teaspoon onion powder

1/4 teaspoon garlic powder

1 teaspoon Celtic sea salt

2 2/3 cups water

INSTRUCTIONS

1. Place parchment paper or dehydrator sheets on two dehydrator trays.
2. Finely mince fresh parsley. Add to large mixing bowl with seeds, salt and spices. Mix until well combined.
3. Spread batter on prepared sheets. Place trays in dehydrator and set to 120 degrees F for 1 hour. Reduce temperature to 105 degrees F for remainder of dehydrating time.
4. After 4 hours dehydrating time, remove trays from dehydrator and use knife to score crackers in preferred shape and size.

Place back in dehydrator and continue dehydrating another 4 hours.

5. Remove trays from dehydrator. Peel crackers from sheets and break apart along score lines. Place crackers directly on dehydrator tray and continue dehydrating another 4 - 12 hours, depending on desired crispness.

6. Remove crackers from dehydrator and serve with your favorite raw dips, spreads and salsas. Or store in an airtight container up to 4 weeks.

Veggie Flax Crackers

Prep Time: 10 minutes

Cook Time: 12 - 24 hours

Servings: 4

INGREDIENTS

1 medium tomato

1 medium onion

2 medium zucchini

1 cup ground flax seed

2 tablespoons coconut aminos (or raw apple cider vinegar)

1/2 teaspoon ground black pepper

1 teaspoon Celtic sea salt

INSTRUCTIONS

1. Place parchment paper or dehydrator sheets on two dehydrator trays.
2. Peel onion and chop. Chop zucchini and tomato. Add to food processor or high-speed blender with flax meal, coconut aminos or vinegar, salt and pepper. Process until well ground, about 2 minutes.
3. Spread batter on prepared sheets. Place trays in dehydrator and set to 120 degrees F for 1 hour. Reduce temperature to 105 degrees F for remainder of dehydrating time.
4. After 4 hours dehydrating time, remove trays from dehydrator and use knife to score crackers in preferred shape and size.

Place back in dehydrator and continue dehydrating another 4 hours.

5. Remove trays from dehydrator. Peel crackers from sheets and break apart along score lines. Place crackers directly on dehydrator tray and continue dehydrating another 4 - 12 hours, depending on desired crispness.

6. Remove crackers from dehydrator and serve with your favorite raw dips, spreads and salsas. Or store in an airtight container up to 4 weeks.

Avocado Cashew Hummus with Cucumber

Prep Time: 5 minutes*

Servings: 4

INGREDIENTS

1 cup raw cashews

1 avocado

Juice of 1/2 lemon

2 garlic cloves

1 teaspoon ground white pepper (or 1/2 teaspoon ground black pepper)

Small bunch fresh cilantro

1/2 teaspoon Celtic sea salt

1 small cucumber

Water

INSTRUCTIONS

1. *Soak cashews in enough water to cover at least 4 hours, or overnight in refrigerator. Drain and rinse.
2. Peel garlic. Juice lemon. Remove cilantro leaves from stem. Add to food processor or high-speed blender with soaked cashews, salt and pepper.
3. Slice avocado in half. Remove pit and scoop flesh into processor. Process until smooth, about 1 - 2 minutes. Add water or raw oil to reach desired consistency, if necessary.
4. Transfer mixture to serving dish.

5. Peel cucumber if desired. Cut diagonally into 1/3 inch slices. Arrange on serving dish.

6. Serve immediately with hummus. Or place in refrigerator for 20 minutes, then serve chilled.

Sundried Tomato Cashew Hummus with Carrots

Prep Time: 5 minutes*

Servings: 4

INGREDIENTS

1 1/2 cup raw cashews

1/4 cup sundried tomatoes

1/4 cup raw tahini (or 1/3 cup raw sesame seeds)

1/2 lemon

1 small garlic clove

1 teaspoon ground white pepper (or 1/2 teaspoon ground black pepper)

1/2 teaspoon Celtic sea salt

2 large carrots

Water

INSTRUCTIONS

1. *Soak cashews in enough water to cover at least 4 hours, or overnight in refrigerator. Drain and rinse.
2. Peel garlic. Juice lemon. Add to food processor or high-speed blender with raw sesame seeds and process until smooth, if using.
3. Or add tahini to processor with soaked cashews, sundried tomatoes, garlic, lemon juice, salt and pepper. Process until smooth, about 1 - 2 minutes. Add water or raw oil to reach desired consistency, if necessary.

4. Transfer mixture to serving dish.
5. Peel carrots if desired. Cut into 4 inch long x 1/2 inch thick sticks. Arrange on serving dish.
6. Serve immediately with hummus. Or place in refrigerator for 20 minutes, then serve chilled.

Cocoa Date Spread

Prep Time: 5 minutes*

Servings: 4

INGREDIENTS

10 - 12 oz dried pitted dates

2 cups water

3 tablespoons raw cocoa powder

1/2 teaspoon ground cinnamon

1/4 teaspoon ground ginger

Ground black pepper, to taste

INSTRUCTIONS

1. *Soak dates in water overnight. Drain and reserve 1/4 cup liquid.

2. Add soaked dates, cocoa powder, cinnamon, ginger and black pepper to taste to food processor or high-speed blender. Pulse until chunky mixture forms. Add reserved liquid to reach desired consistency, if necessary.

3. Or add dates to medium mixing bowl with cocoa powder, cinnamon, ginger and black pepper to taste. Mash with large fork or potato masher for about 5 minutes, until chunky mixture forms. Add reserved liquid to reach desired consistency, if necessary.

4. Transfer to serving dish and serve with fruits, veggies, or raw crackers and breads.

Cashew Spinach Dip with Bell Pepper

Prep Time: 10 minutes

Servings: 2

INGREDIENTS

2 - 3 cups spinach leaves

1 1/2 cups raw cashews

3 garlic cloves

1 lemon

1/3 cup water

1/4 teaspoon mustard powder (or mustard seeds)

1/2 teaspoon ground white pepper (or 1/4 teaspoon ground black pepper)

1/2 teaspoon Celtic sea salt

1 red bell pepper

INSTRUCTIONS

1. Cut bell pepper in half and remove seeds, veins and stems. Slice peppers into 1 - 1 1/2 inch strips. Arrange on serving dish and set aside.

2. Juice lemon. Peel garlic. Add to food processor or high-speed blender with cashews and mustard powder or seeds. Process until finely ground, about 2 minutes.

3. Add salt, pepper and water. Process until smooth. Add spinach and pulse until spinach is desired texture.

4. Transfer mixture to serving dish. Serving immediately with bell pepper slices. Or refrigerate 20 minutes and serve chilled.

Chocolate Hazelnut Spread with Apples

Prep Time: 5 minutes*

Servings: 2

INGREDIENTS

1 cup raw hazelnuts

1/4 cup raw cocoa powder

1/4 cup raw honey (or dried pitted dates)

2/3 teaspoon vanilla

1/4 teaspoon Celtic sea salt

2 apples

Raw nut milk (optional)

Water

INSTRUCTIONS

1. *Soak hazelnuts in enough water to cover overnight in refrigerator. Soak dates in enough water to cover overnight in refrigerator, if using. Drain and rinse.

2. Add soaked hazelnuts to food processor or high-speed blender and process until smooth, up to 10 minutes. Scrape down sides as needed.

3. Add honey or soaked dates, cocoa powder, vanilla and salt. Process until smooth, about 1 minute. Add nut milk to reach desired consistency, if necessary.

4. Transfer mixture to serving dish.

5. Remove core, seeds and stems from apples. Slice into wedges and arrange on serving dish. Serve immediately.

Cashew Butter Date Snacks

Prep Time: 5 minutes

Servings: 2

INGREDIENTS

6 whole dried pitted dates

Pinch ground cinnamon

Raw Cashew Butter

1 cup raw cashews

1 dried pitted date

1 teaspoon raw oil (coconut, walnut, almond, sesame, etc.)

1/2 teaspoon ground cinnamon

1/4 teaspoon Celtic sea salt

(or 1/2 cup prepared raw cashew butter)

INSTRUCTIONS

1. For *Cashew Butter*, add cashews, date, cinnamon, salt and oil to food processor or high-speed blender. Process until smooth, up to 5 minutes. Let mixture rest between periods of processing to reach desired consistency, if necessary.

2. Slice dates in half lengthwise. Use small spoon to fill date halves with prepared or *Raw Cashew Butter*. Sprinkle ground cinnamon over filled dates.

3. Arrange on serving dish and serve immediately.

Very Cherry Energy Bars

Prep Time: 25 minutes

Servings: 6

INGREDIENTS

1 cup dried cherries

1/4 cup dried pitted dates

1 cup raw almonds

1/4 teaspoon ground cinnamon

1/4 teaspoon vanilla

1/8 teaspoon Celtic sea salt

1/3 cup warm water

1/2 sour orange (or orange or tangerine)

INSTRUCTIONS

1. Zest and juice orange into small mixing bowl. Add warm water and dried cherries. Toss to coat and set aside 10 minutes.

2. Line loaf pan with parchment paper.

3. Add nuts and dates to food processor or high-speed blender. Drain soaked cherries and add to processor with cinnamon, vanilla and salt. Process for about 1 minute, until mixture is coarsely ground and sticks together when pressed.

4. Scrape mixture into prepared loaf pan and press firmly into bottom with hands or spatula.

5. Place in refrigerator and chill for 10 minutes. Remove and cut into 6 bars.

6. Serve immediately. Or store in refrigerator up to 2 weeks.

Sweet Coconut Ambrosia Salad

Prep Time: 15 minutes*

Servings: 2

INGREDIENTS

3 mature coconuts

1 1/2 cups water

6 clementines or tangerines (about 1 cup segments)

1 cup fresh pineapple (chopped)

1 cup pecans (chopped)

1 cup fresh cherries (pitted)

INSTRUCTIONS

1. Remove coconut flesh from shells. Add 1 coconut and water to food processor or high-speed blender. Process until well blended and fairly smooth, about 1 - 2 minutes.

2. Strain mixture through nut milk bag, cheesecloth or strainer into container. Add coconut milk back to blender with flesh of 2nd coconut. Process again until well blended and thick, about 1 - 2 minutes.

3. Strain mixture through nut milk bag, cheesecloth or strainer into container. Reserve pulp and set aside to dry and dehydrate, then use as coconut flour.

4. *For thicker coconut cream, set aside thickened milk in refrigerator about 20 minutes and allow fat to separate. Remove coconut cream from refrigerator and scoop out risen fat into medium mixing bowl.

5. Or add coconut cream milk to medium mixing bowl. Peel oranges or tangerines and remove segments. Peel pineapple and chop. Cut cherries in half and pit. Chop pecans. Add to coconut cream.

6. Add remaining coconut flesh to clean food processor with shredding attachment and process, or grate with grater. Add coconut to mixture. Stir to combine.

7. Cover mixture and place in refrigerator for 2 hours. Remove and transfer to serving dishes.

8. Serve chilled.

Sweet Carrot Raisin Salad

Prep Time: 5 minutes

Servings: 2

INSTRUCTIONS

2 large carrots

2 tablespoons red raisins

2 tablespoons golden raisins

1/4 cup raw slivered almonds (or sliced almonds)

1/2 small orange (or tangerine)

1/4 teaspoon ground cinnamon

DIRECTIONS

1. Add carrots to food processor with shredding attachment and process, or grate with grater. Add to medium mixing bowl with raisins, almonds and cinnamon.

2. Zest *then* juice orange. Add to carrot mixture and toss to combine.

3. Transfer to serving dishes and serve immediately. Or refrigerate 20 minutes and serve chilled.

Sweet Coconut Rice with Mango

Prep Time: 10 minutes*

Servings: 2

INSTRUCTIONS

1 fresh coconut (or 2/3 cup desiccated, shredded or flaked coconut)

1/4 cup raw honey (or 1/4 cup dried pitted dates)

1/4 teaspoon ground ginger(or 1/4 inch piece fresh ginger)

1 mango

INGREDIENTS

1. *Soak dried coconut and dried pitted dates in enough water to cover overnight in refrigerator, if using. Drain coconut and add to medium mixing bowl. Drain dates and reserve 2 tablespoons soaking liquid.

2. Or remove fresh coconut flesh from shell and add to food processor with shredding attachment and process, or grate with grater. Add to medium mixing bowl.

3. Add soaked dates and soaking liquid to clean food processor or high-speed and process until smooth, if using.

4. Peel fresh ginger and mince or finely grate, if using. Add raw honey or date purée to shredded coconut with ground or fresh ginger. Mix to combine. Transfer to serving dishes.

5. Slice mango in half around pit. Remove peel and dice or thinly slice flesh. Add over sweet shredded coconut.

6. Serve immediately. Or refrigerate 20 minutes and serve chilled.

Sweet Almond Crunch Cookies

Prep Time: 20 minutes

Servings: 12

INGREDIENTS

3/4 cup raw almond butter (or 1 cup raw almonds)

2 - 4 tablespoons raw honey (or 1/4 cup dried pitted dates)

1 tablespoon ground chia seed or flax meal (or whole seeds)

1 teaspoon cinnamon

1/2 teaspoon Celtic sea salt

1/4 cup raw almonds

INSTRUCTIONS

1. Line baking dish with parchment paper.
2. Add 1/4 cup raw almonds to food processor or high-speed blender and process until finely chopped. Set aside.
3. Add whole chia or flax seeds to high-speed blender or spice grinder and grind to fine powder, if using.
4. Add chia or flax meal to food processor or high-speed blender with remaining almonds or almond butter, honey or dates, cinnamon and salt. Process until smooth, thick paste forms, up to 5 minutes. Let mixture rest between periods of processing to reach desired consistency, if necessary.
5. Spread mixture in parchment lined dish. Place in refrigerator or freezer for 10 minutes.
6. Remove dish and scoop with tablespoon or melon baller. Roll into balls with hands.

7. Place chopped almonds in shallow dish and roll balls in almonds to coat.

8. Transfer coated almond cookies to serving dish. Serve immediately. Or refrigerate 20 minutes and serve chilled.

Chewy Ginger Cookies

Prep Time: 20 minutes*

Servings: 12

INGREDIENTS

1/2 cup raw cashews (frozen)

1 1/2 cups dried pitted dates (1 cup chopped)

2 inch piece fresh ginger

1 teaspoon ground ginger

1/4 teaspoon ground cinnamon

1/2 cup unsweetened flaked or shredded coconut

INSTRUCTIONS

1. Place cashews in freezer for a few hours to overnight.
2. Add frozen nuts to food processor or high-speed blender. Pulse until coarsely ground.
3. Peel and finely grate fresh ginger. Add to processor with dates, ground ginger and cinnamon. Process until mixture is well broken down and sticks together.
4. Form mixture into 12 balls. Add coconut flakes to shallow dish. Roll balla in coconut until well coated, then gently press to flatten slightly.
5. Arrange on serving dish and cover. Place in freezer for at least 10 minutes, until set up and firm.
6. Remove from freezer and serve chilled. Or store in freezer or refrigerator.

Chocolate Dusted Almonds

Prep Time: 20 minutes*

Servings: 2

INGREDIENTS

1 cup raw almonds

1 tablespoon raw cocoa powder

1 tablespoon raw honey

1/8 teaspoon ground cinnamon

1/8 teaspoon vanilla

INSTRUCTIONS

1. Add almonds and honey to small mixing bowl and toss to combine.
2. Add cocoa, cinnamon and vanilla and toss to evenly coat.
3. Transfer to serving dish and serve immediately.

Chocolate Chia Pudding

Prep Time: 15 minutes

Servings: 2

INGREDIENTS

1 cup nut milk (or 2 mature coconuts + 1 1/2 cups water)

2 - 4 tablespoons raw honey (or dried pitted dates)

2 - 4 tablespoons whole chia seeds

2 - 3 tablespoons cocoa powder

1/2 teaspoon vanilla

INSTRUCTIONS

1. Remove coconut flesh from shells. Add 1 coconut and water to food processor or high-speed blender. Process until well blended and fairly smooth, about 1- 2 minutes.

2. Strain mixture through nut milk bag, cheesecloth or strainer into container. Add coconut milk back to blender with remaining coconut flesh. Process again until well blended and fairly smooth, about 1 minute.

3. Strain mixture through nut milk bag, cheesecloth or strainer into container. Reserve pulp and set aside to dry and dehydrate, then use as coconut flour.

4. Add nut milk to high-speed blender with dates and process until smooth, if using.

5. Or add nut milk to small mixing bowl with honey or stevia, cocoa powder, vanilla and chia seeds. Whisk to combine. Set aside to thicken, about 1 minute.

6. Pour mixture into serving dishes and serve immediately. Or refrigerate 20 minutes and serve chilled.

Coconut Rice Pudding

Prep Time: 20 minutes

Servings: 4

INGREDIENTS

3 fresh coconuts (or 2 cups unsweetened flaked or shredded coconut)

1 cup water

1/4 - 1/2 cup raw honey (or dried pitted dates)

1 teaspoon vanilla

Water

INSTRUCTIONS

1. *Soak 1 1/2 cups flaked coconut and dates in enough water to cover in refrigerator overnight. Then drain, if using.

2. Or remove fresh coconut flesh from shells.

3. Add flesh of 1 fresh coconut or 3/4 cup soaked coconut, and water to high-speed blender. Process until well blended and fairly smooth, about 1- 2 minutes.

4. Strain mixture through nut milk bag, cheesecloth or strainer into container. Add coconut milk back to blender with flesh of 1 fresh coconut or remaining soaked coconut. Process again until well blended and fairly smooth, about 1 minute.

5. Strain mixture through nut milk bag, cheesecloth or strainer into container. Reserve pulp and set aside to dry and dehydrate, then use as coconut flour.

6. Add coconut cream, soaked dates and vanilla to food processor or high-speed blender. Process until smooth, about 1 minute.

7. Or add coconut cream to medium mixing bowl with raw honey and vanilla.
8. Add remaining fresh coconut flesh to food processer with shredding attachment and process, or shred with grater.
9. Add shredded fresh coconut or flaked coconut to coconut cream mixture and whisk until well combined.
10. Pour into serving dishes and serve immediately. Or refrigerate for 20 minutes and serve chilled.

Nori with Almond Cheese

Prep Time: 15 minutes*

Servings: 2

INGREDIENTS

4 - 6 sheets dried nori (seaweed paper)

Almond cheese

1 cup raw almonds

2 tablespoons raw oil (coconut, walnut, almond, sesame, etc.)

2 tablespoons lemon juice (or raw apple cider vinegar)

1 garlic clove

1/4 teaspoon paprika

1/4 teaspoon ground white pepper (or ground black pepper)

1/2 teaspoon Celtic sea salt

Water

INSTRUCTIONS

1. *For *Almond Cheese*, soak almonds in enough water to cover overnight. Drain and rinse. Pop off skins and discard.

2. Peel garlic and add to food processor or high-speed blender with soaked almonds, oil, lemon juice and/or vinegar, salt and spices. Process until smooth, about 2 minutes. Add water to reach desired consistency, if necessary.

3. Transfer mixture to small serving dish. Cut nori into small sheets and arrange on serving dish.

4. Serve immediately. Or refrigerate for 20 minutes and serve chilled.

Quick Asian Slaw

Prep Time: 15 minutes*

Servings: 4

INGREDIENTS

1/2 head red cabbage (2 cups shredded)

2 broccoli stalks (2 cups shredded)

1/4 cup dried cranberries

1/4 cup raw sliced or slivered almonds

2 tablespoons raw sunflower seeds

2 green onions (scallions)

1 carrot

1 lemon

1/2 orange

2 tablespoons raw honey

2 tablespoons raw sesame oil (or coconut, walnut, almond oil, etc.)

2 tablespoons apple cider vinegar

1/2 teaspoon ground ginger

1 teaspoon ground white pepper (or black pepper)

1 teaspoon Celtic sea salt

INSTRUCTIONS

1. Add broccoli and carrot to food processor with shredding attachment, or grate with grater. Slice green onions. Shred cabbage. Add to large mixing bowl.

2. Add cranberries, almonds, sunflower seeds, honey, oil, vinegar, ginger, salt, pepper and squeeze of lemon and orange. Mix until well combined.
3. *Transfer mixture and for 90 minutes. Serve chilled.

Awesome Strawberry Salsa

Prep Time: 5 minutes*

Servings: 4

INGREDIENTS

2 cups fresh strawberries

1/2 small white onion

1/4 red bell pepper

Medium bunch fresh mint

1/2 lime

1/2 orange

1/2 teaspoon ground black pepper

INSTRUCTIONS

1. Remove strawberry stems and leaves, then finely dice. Add to medium mixing bowl.

2. Peel onion and finely dice. Remove mint leave s from stem then chiffon, or thinly slice. Add to strawberries with pepper and squeeze of lime and orange. Mix until well combined.

3. Transfer mixture to serving dish and serve immediately with raw chips. Or refrigerate for 20 minutes and serve chilled.

Supreme Mango Salsa

Prep Time: 10 minutes

Servings: 4

INGREDIENTS

2 mangos

1/4 small red onion

1/4 red bell pepper

Small bunch fresh cilantro

1 lime

1/2 fresh jalapeño pepper

1/4 teaspoon Celtic sea salt

INSTRUCTIONS

1. Slice mangos in half around pit. Remove peel and finely dice flesh. Add to medium mixing bowl.

2. Peel onion and dice. Remove seeds, stem and vein from bell pepper, then finely dice. Finely chop cilantro. Remove seeds and stem from jalapeño, then mince. Add to mango with salt and squeeze of lime. Mix until well combined

3. Transfer mixture to serving dish and serve immediately with raw chips. Or refrigerate for 20 minutes and serve chilled.

Hot Apricot Pineapple Salsa

Prep Time: 15 minutes

Servings: 4

INGREDIENTS

1 cup fresh pineapple (diced)

3 fresh apricots

1/2 green bell pepper

1/2 cup cherry tomatoes

2 shallots

2 garlic cloves

1 lime

1 fresh Serrano pepper

Small bunch cilantro leaves

1/2 teaspoon cayenne pepper

1/4 teaspoon Celtic sea salt

INSTRUCTIONS

1. Peel pineapple and finely dice. Cut apricots in half and remove pits, then finely dice. Add to medium mixing bowl.

2. Peel shallots and thinly slice. Peel garlic and mince or thinly slice. Remove seeds, stem and vein from bell pepper, then finely dice. Quarter cherry tomatoes. Add to pineapple and apricot.

3. Finely chop cilantro. Remove seeds and stem from Serrano pepper, then mince. Add to bowl with salt, cayenne and squeeze of lime. Mix until well combined.

4. Transfer mixture to serving dish and serve immediately with raw chips. Or refrigerate for 20 minutes and serve chilled.

Fresh Zesty Pico de Gallo

Prep Time: 15 minutes*

Servings: 4

INGREDIENTS

4 plum tomatoes

1/2 small red onion

Small bunch fresh cilantro

1/2 jalapeño pepper

1/2 lime

1 garlic clove

1/8 teaspoon garlic powder

1/4 teaspoon ground cumin

1/4 teaspoon Celtic sea salt

1/4 teaspoon ground black pepper

INSTRUCTIONS

1. Finely dice tomatoes. Peel and dice onion. Add to medium mixing bowl.
2. Finely chop cilantro. Remove seeds, veins and stem from jalapeño, then mince. Peel and mince garlic. Add to tomatoes with salt, spices and squeeze of lime. Mix until well combined.
3. Transfer mixture to serving dish
4. *Refrigerate 3 hours. Serve room temperature or chilled with raw chips.

Holy Loaded Guacamole

Prep Time: 5 minutes

Servings: 2

INGREDIENTS

2 ripe avocados

1 small plum tomato

1/4 small red onion

Medium bunch fresh cilantro

1/2 lime

1/2 teaspoon smoked paprika

1/2 teaspoon ground black pepper

1/2 teaspoon Celtic sea salt

INSTRUCTIONS

1. Cut avocados in half and remove pits. Scoop flesh into small mixing bowl.
2. Peel onion and dice. Dice tomato. Finely chop cilantro. Add to avocado with salt, spices, and squeeze of lime. Mash with fork until well combined.
3. Transfer mixture to serving dish and serve immediately with raw chips. Or refrigerate for 20 minutes and serve chilled.

Spicy Stuffed Jalapeños

Prep Time: 15 minutes*

Dehydrating Time: 8 - 24 hours

Servings: 4

INGREDIENTS

6 fresh jalapeño peppers

1 cup raw sunflower seeds

1/2 cup water

1/4 cup nutritional yeast

1 lemon

2 teaspoons onion powder

1/2 teaspoon cayenne pepper

1 teaspoon Celtic sea salt

Water

INSTRUCTIONS

1. *Soak sunflower seeds in enough water to cover for 2 hours. Drain and rinse.

2. Cut jalapeños in half lengthwise and remove stems, seeds and veins. Place peppers on dehydrator tray.

3. Juice lemon. Add to food processor or high-speed blender with soaked sunflower seeds, water, nutritional yeast, salt, pepper and spices. Process until thick, smooth paste forms, about 2 minutes.

4. Fill piping bag with mixture and pipe into jalapeño halves. Or use teaspoon to scoop filling into jalapeño halves.

5. Place stuffed peppers on dehydrator sheets filling-side up. Set dehydrator to 110 degrees F for 8 - 24 hours, depending on desired texture.

6. Remove peppers from dehydrator and serve immediately.

www.ingramcontent.com/pod-product-compliance
Lightning Source LLC
Chambersburg PA
CBHW070104290526
45789CB00005B/1913